AIM TRUE

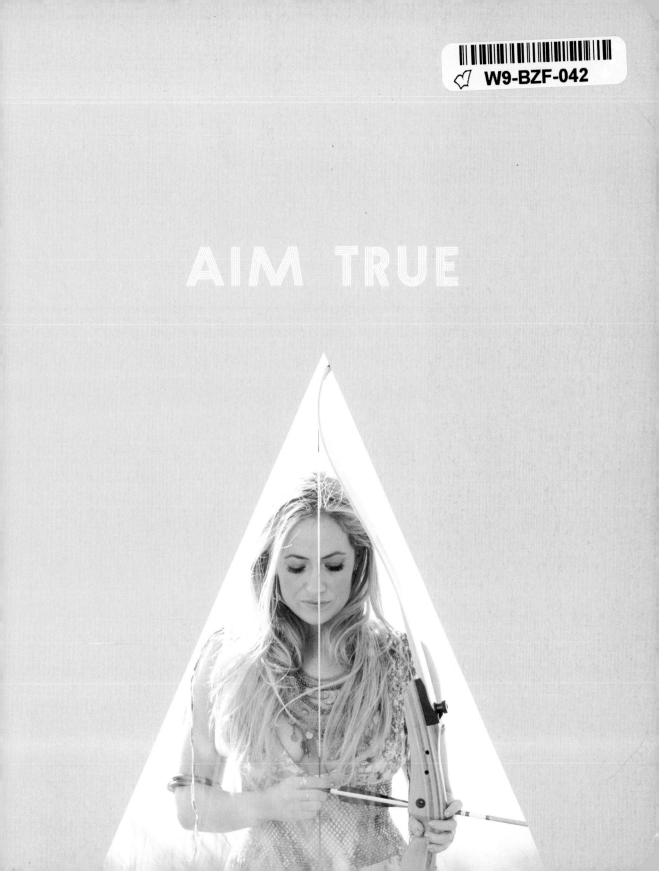

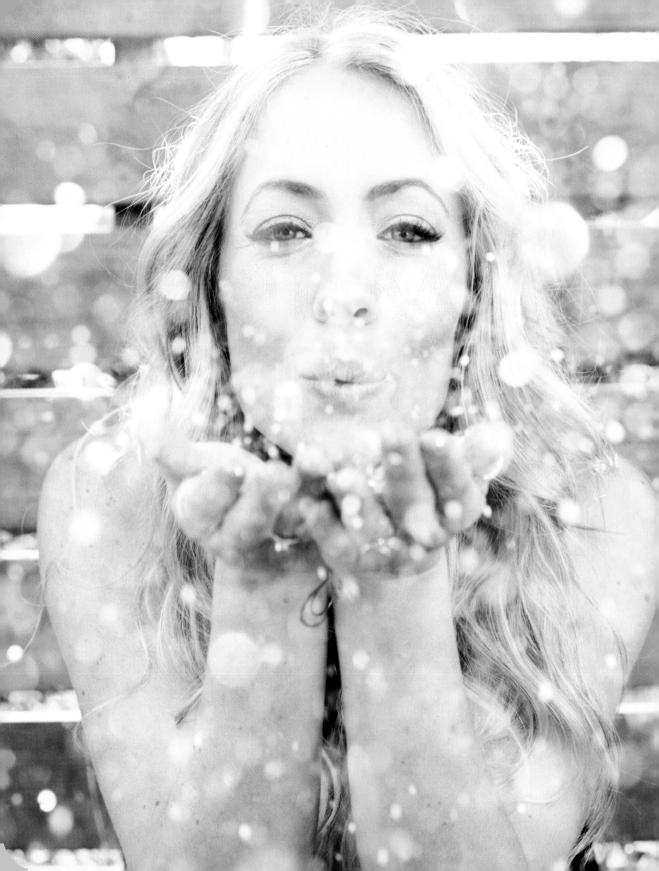

Advance Praise for
Kathryn Budig and *Aim True*

"Kathryn Budig is a transformational leader, rockstar yogi, and an inspiring force in the world. Her work touches thousands of people worldwide."

> — Gabrielle Bernstein, *New York Times* bestselling author

"It is a blessing and a treat to escape into Kathryn's world. Her teaching is restorative to my mind, body, and soul."

> — Blake Mycoskie, founder, Toms Shoes

"Kathryn has helped me add strength and flexibility to my body, especially after having a baby, with fun and personalized workouts. I look forward to our sessions and feeling great about my body!"

> — Giada De Laurentiis, Food Network host

"The yoga practice Kathryn Budig taught me both strengthened me and made me a better performer. Kathryn rocks."

> — Melissa Etheridge, singer

AIM TRUE

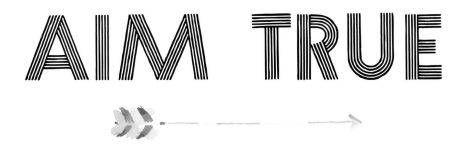

Love Your Body, Eat Without Fear,
Nourish Your Spirit, Discover True Balance!

Kathryn Budig

𝒲𝓂

WILLIAM MORROW

An Imprint of HarperCollinsPublishers

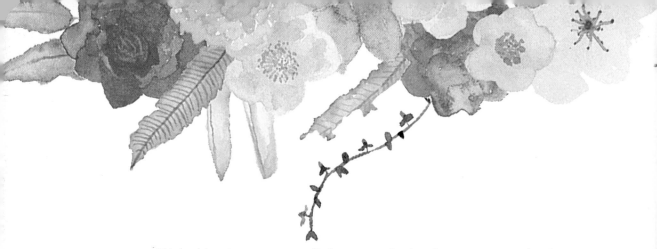

This book is written as a source of information only. The information contained in this book should by no means be considered a substitute for the advice of a qualified medical professional, who should always be consulted before beginning any new diet, exercise, or other health program. All efforts have been made to ensure the accuracy of the information contained in this book as of the date published. The author, publisher, and contributors expressly disclaim responsibility for any adverse effects arising from the use or application of the information contained herein.

HarperCollins books may be purchased for educational, business, or sales promotional use. For information please e-mail the Special Markets Department at SPsales @harpercollins.com.

FIRST EDITION

Designed by Leah Carlson-Stanisic

Photography by Cheyenne Ellis and Lesley Unruh

Food styling by Cynthia Groseclose

Prop styling by Kenneth Hyatt, Justin Schram, and Nicolette Owen

Beauty styling by Sabra Mizzell

Illustrations by Elissa Genello

Chapter 5 contributions by Deborah Kim

Photo on page 257 by Jasper Johal for ToeSox

Moon art on page xii by runLenarun/Shutterstock, Inc

Watercolor art on page xii by solarbird/Shutterstock, Inc

Library of Congress Cataloging-in-Publication Data has been applied for.

ISBN 978-0-06-241971-2

16 17 18 19 20 OV/RRD 10 9 8 7 6 5 4 3 2 1

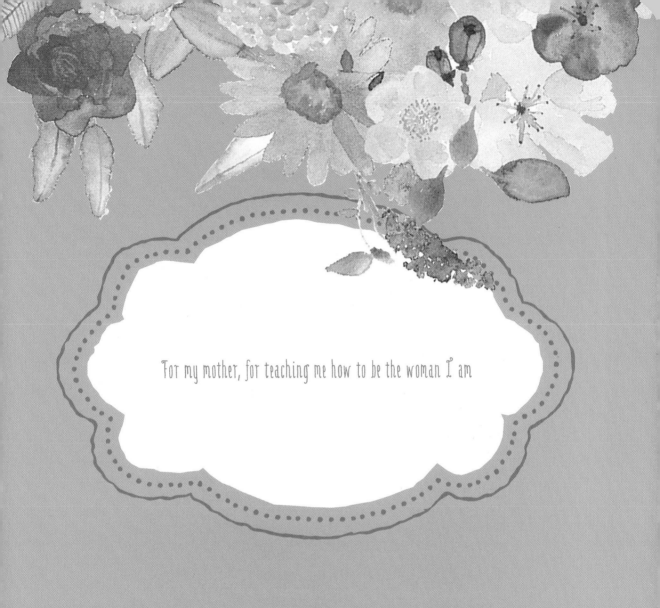

For my mother, for teaching me how to be the woman I am

CONTENTS

Nourish Your Spirit

Discover True Balance

AIM TRUE

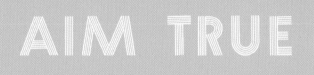

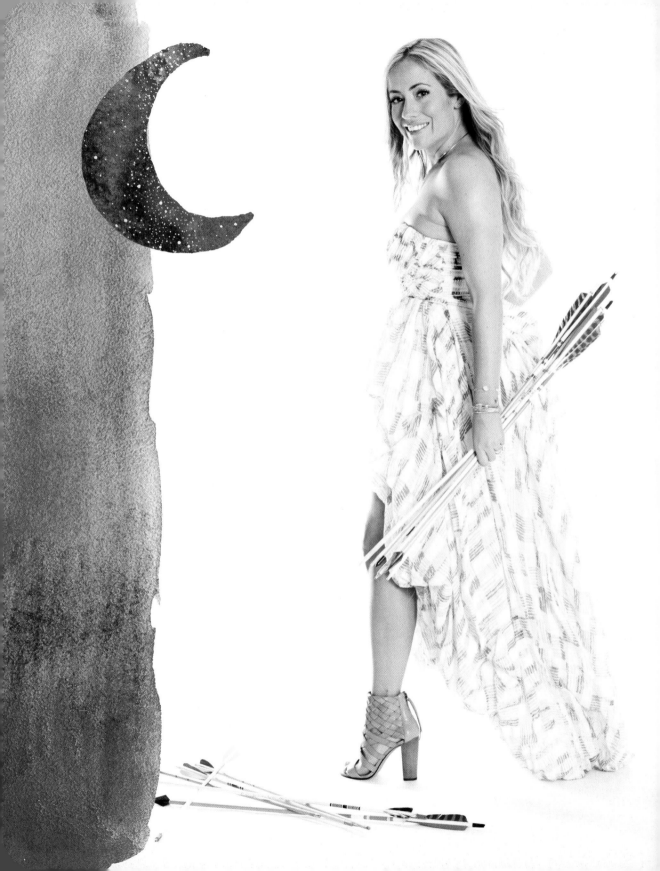

INTRODUCTION

*E*ach of us will have our own reaction to the words *aim true*. The phrase generally means that we're going in the right direction, that our path is correct, and our choices are well made. If I were to ask a group of people to give me a definition of "aim true," they could easily come up with an agreed collective statement, yet each will have a unique definition. That's the beauty of aiming true—it's universal and personal all in the same breath. As you journey through these pages, my hope is that each word will bring you closer to your own definition of what it means to aim true—a verbal tattoo that lives in your heart, showing how you want to live your life.

Aim true is my own personal mantra. I grew up in Kansas. It was a beautiful place in time where cell phones did not exist and I could be let out to play as long as I was home for dinner. I absolutely adored it. I spent hours inspecting plants, sucking out drops of sweetness from honeysuckles, feasting on mulberries, and creating armies of snails. Those days spent outside were fueled by my imagination and love for anything magical and epic. I would play Robin Hood and the full cast of characters all by myself, swinging from tree limbs and rolling down hills. I also developed an early love for ancient Greek mythology. I knew all of the gods and goddesses, demigods, titans, and monsters. Being a tomboy, I had a particular fondness for one goddess in particular.

Artemis.

Artemis (or Diana, in the Roman tradition) was known as the goddess of the moon and the hunt, and the protector of women. All of this appealed to me at the tender age of eight, as my other option was Aphrodite, and she liked boys. Ew.

My girl Artemis was the one who went to her father Zeus and told him she knew she was different. She had no desire to marry, but rather wanted to spend her life with her tribe of sisters in the woods where she could hunt, be in nature, and fully be herself. He granted her this, and off she went. In artwork, Artemis is always depicted bearing the crescent moon on her forehead, wearing a knee-length tunic, and carrying her bow and quiver of arrows. She marched to the beat of her own drum, and I admired her for that. I couldn't really understand how deep this admiration would go until years later, during another chapter of my life story . . .

I had been living in Los Angeles for years, and daydreaming had been replaced with day-to-day life management, like paying taxes. There was not a trace of Artemis or magical living on my mind. In fact, I had been dragging myself through the coals of the completely magicless dating scene. After being broken up with by what felt like Boyfriend #86, I had reached a point of desperation where I didn't care about Prince Charming anymore—I just wanted somebody, anybody, to love me. What's worse than being broken up with by someone you adore? That's right—someone you don't. I was feeling particularly pathetic one day when I received a phone call from a fellow yoga teacher telling me she had just started to date the guy who had dumped me.

Let's just add salt to the wound.

I took a deep breath and listened. I'm a yoga teacher, after all. I've been trained to accept honestly, to be nonreactive and open to all. Which I did to my best ability, then hung up and made a detour to go do what I do best when I'm upset—shop.

I pulled up to my favorite local boutique and stormed in with a mission. I ransacked the store only to land in front of the jewelry section, where they had a display of charm necklaces. I browsed through the selection and stopped at the sight of a gold arrow dangling nicely next to a gold crescent moon. These powerful Artemis images opened a floodgate to my childhood memories that I had completely forgotten. Memories of being completely happy and fulfilled by myself and my imagination.

Aim True

This moment struck me in the head like a frying pan. I decided to buy the necklace, but in particular, to wear the gold arrow around my neck every single day as a reminder that I am whole, I am complete, and I am very much in charge of my own happiness.

I walked out of that store revived and with purpose. Anytime I felt ready to throw myself a pity party, instead I would simply touch the necklace as a reminder of my strength. I mean, what would Artemis do if a guy broke up with her? Sit around and cry? No, she'd pull out one of her arrows and move on!

So move on I did. Within weeks, I was feeling so much better I started to wonder—was there actual power behind this necklace? Was I reconnecting with a long-lost energy from my childhood that had protected me? What was going on here?

I sat down at my computer and started to research the goddess Artemis. I reread her stories, admired the paintings and sculptures, and stumbled upon a prayer written to her.

Artemis, goddess of the moon, make my aim true.

A trail of goose bumps appeared on my arms. I continued to read:

Give me goals to seek, and the constant means and determination to achieve them.

This was the beginning. I could feel it. I knew what it meant to have goals and determination, but in that moment, I also discovered that if I wanted to achieve them, I first had to aim true. I took a deep breath and realized, *The work starts now. To determine what it means to aim true will change my life.* Challenge accepted.

Are you ready to discover what *aim true* means to you?

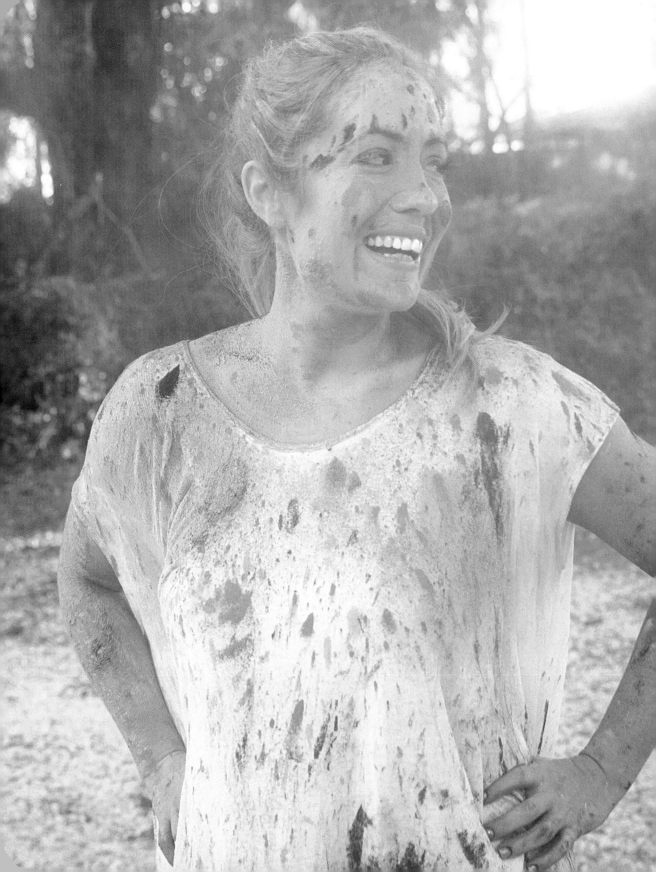

Love Your Body

DON'T ASK YOURSELF WHAT THE WORLD NEEDS.
ASK YOURSELF WHAT MAKES YOU COME
ALIVE AND THEN GO DO THAT.
BECAUSE WHAT THE WORLD NEEDS IS PEOPLE
WHO HAVE COME ALIVE.

—Howard Thurman, as told to Gil Bailie

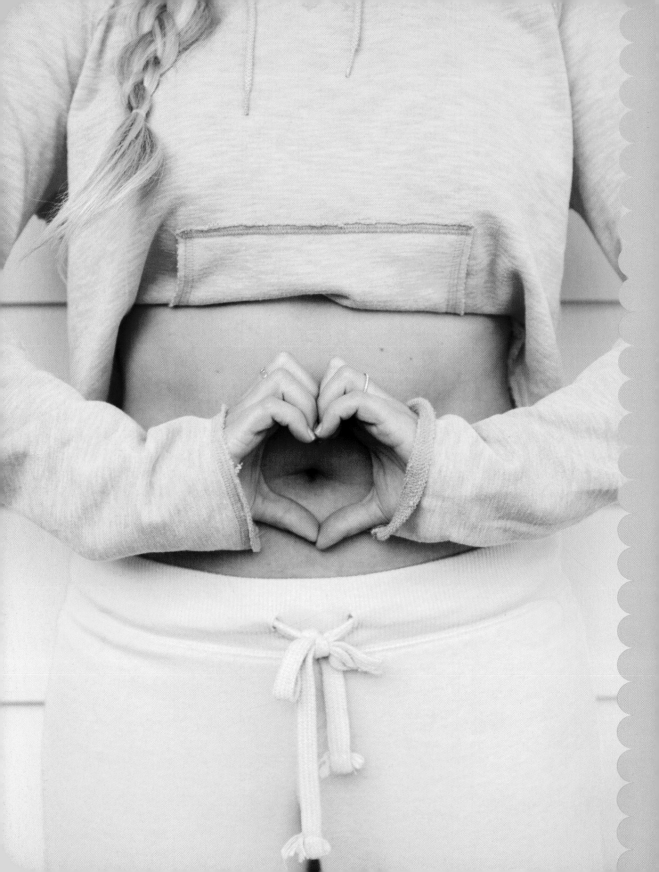

One

LOVE WHO *You* *Are* RIGHT NOW

*Y*ou are fantastic. A unique being tackling this incredibly juicy human experience that is riddled with challenges, miracles, mysteries, and questions that guide and inspire your path. As someone with the desire to aim true, you know you're reading this book as an opportunity to embrace your talents and find a peaceful state of self-acceptance. Many health or lifestyle books like to point out what's *wrong* with you. They'll address where you've gone astray, and then give you a long list of chores and ways to fix yourself.

Let me make something abundantly clear: there is nothing wrong with you! You are a fully equipped dream weaver who makes magic reality with your toolbox full of experiences and passion. Every laugh line on your face tells a story, any scar displays your strength, and stretch marks are code for growth and willingness to evolve and change.

In fact, we are all *perfectly imperfect*, like Mona here. The Japanese call this *wabi-sabi*—the acceptance of transience and imperfection. This doesn't mean you take a big sigh and accept the cards you've been given with dismay. It means you play whatever cards you've been dealt with finesse and austerity. We continue to grow every day because of our individual and collective life experiences. Our perceived flaws, whether physical or emotional, are what make us unique. *Strong* doesn't mean "fitting media's version of healthy." *Beauty* doesn't mean "flawless and eternally young." *Smart* doesn't mean "making safe choices." The world doesn't need an army of Barbies and Kens. We need crooked smiles that show our humor, loud laughs that stem from the belly, and crazy, innovative ideas to save us from the safe but monotonous norm.

It's easy to forget to take pride in who we are when we've become habituated to focus on what's come before or what's next. This can be in our own life (in the form of past relationships or future jobs) or the lives and events surrounding us in person and in our digital lives (in the form of that person on the mat next to you acing a pose or that digital friend who always seems to be three steps ahead of you in terms of life goals). Regardless of these emotions triggered on your walk down memory lane or looking ahead, understand that you wouldn't be *you* without those experiences. Every experience is an opportunity to grow.

Along this journey, there will be tears of joy and hot springs of pain, but they all count and make us the wiser. Instead of focusing on perfecting ourselves, let's focus on what makes us shine.

What Makes You Come Alive?

I tend to get two distinct reactions from people when I ask this question in the workshops I teach around the world. The first type of person rattles off a list like a four-year-old ordering at an ice cream shop:

> *"I love my dog! My family is the center of my universe! I can't wait to practice yoga every day! I get seriously emotional over professional baseball!"*

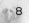

The other type of person looks at me with wide, puppy-dog eyes and a shrug of the shoulders after coming back answerless.

The truth is, knowing what makes you come alive isn't the easiest thing to know or understand. We're here to figure that out together. Some of us are deeply aware of what we're passionate about, while others may feel like they're just trying to stay alive one day at a time, fighting the daily grind of life. To repeat the first lines of the Artemis prayer, "make my aim true. Give me goals to seek and the constant means and determination to achieve them." If we want to get to these so-called "goals," we need to make our aims true. The first step toward this is working to understand what gifts you have to offer the world. Your natural talents and innate gifts—when understood and used daily—are part of what makes you come alive. Once we know what makes our heart beat, it's easier to understand what goals matter to us versus the ones that we may have been working toward mindlessly.

GET HONEST WITH YOURSELF: START A JOURNAL

As you begin to consider this first question of the journey, I'd love for you to keep a journal where you can write down answers, thoughts, inspiration, and anything that comes up for you as you continue to read this book. Owning your feelings is a step toward figuring out what makes you come alive. When something in these pages inspires you or shakes you up—write it down. It may not even seem that important or even logical at the time, but it takes time to put together a complex puzzle. Every piece counts. The key to journaling is: keep it real! Be honest with yourself, even if it's embarrassing and unpleasant. Let this journal be a safe place where you can express yourself freely without any fear of judgment.

I have a few more questions I'd like you to answer for yourself:

What are your talents + unique qualities?

Write down at least five amazing qualities that you possess. What are your talents? What makes you uniquely you? You can write things down like "I make the best pasta sauce in the world, and friends are constantly banging down my door to get me to feed them" or "Every time my friends are feeling upset, they call me because I'm an amazing, unbiased listener." Perhaps it's something physical like "My alignment in downward-facing dog is so beautiful it makes my teacher cry." The point of this exercise is to understand that unique qualities and talents range from the physical to the emotional to the spiritual.

It can take some time getting used to saying why we're so amazing because we've been trained to think that saying fantastic things about ourselves is narcissistic. But there is nothing narcissistic about knowing and acknowledging why you're special. In fact, if you don't know what makes you brilliant, you're performing a "sayonara fishy" flush of your birthright traits that are your *duty* to share with the world. A huge part of aiming true is pursuing what makes your heart beat and letting your light shine. We must know what our talents are in order to properly explore the goals that fit our path.

Still struggling to come up with your list of five? Imagine I were to sit down and interview your best friend about you. I'd ask them, "Why is _____ your best friend?" To which they'd easily rattle off a long list of reasons. Try to see your beauty through someone else's eyes. My hope is that, with time and practice, you'll be able to feel and commit to your talent in the first person.

What fills you up? What tears you apart?

These next two questions are closely linked. Your passion is often quite similar to what pulls at your heartstrings. For example, I am passionate about empowering people to fully love themselves and live big. I want them to shine in hopes that they can influence others to live

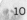

in the same way. Flip the coin, and it breaks my heart to see people live small, to see talented people lose hope and tell themselves they are useless. We all have talents—they lie in accessing your own unique gifts. That means waking up to what you're excited about pursuing. So you see, my heartache and my passion are closely connected. Your answers to these two questions can guide you in the process of finding what makes you come alive.

What would you do if there was no chance of failing?

This might be my favorite question. Consider what you would do if you could do *anything* with your life—live anywhere, have any type of job, be with anyone you want. Let your imagination go wild! Write up your "dream" life, and here's the catch (and remember the key to journaling as mentioned on page 9): don't edit yourself. These words and dreams are just for you. Don't let past experiences or the judgment of others stop you. Write as if you have zero chance of failing and every opportunity granted. Strip your mind of all the comments or experiences that have prevented you from feeling good enough, smart enough, or strong enough. Go back to your heart and ask it what it really wants. Allowing your heart to speak freely without the highly opinionated mind interrupting is like strapping on your ruby slippers and following the yellow brick road to creating change in your life.

What has been stopping you in your tracks?

We're accumulating a good list of qualities, passions, and dreams to inspire and keep us driven, but what about the experiences and feelings we cling to that may be holding us back? Past experiences are deeply powerful and can be difficult to move beyond—from unresolved stories to painful statements uttered by influential people that create an unpleasant echo for life. We have to be so incredibly careful with the words we share, because they have the ability to scar as well as to empower.

In my past life (or so it seems), I was a musical theater actress. I was a trained singer who had a flair for the dramatic and was instructed to use vibrato when I sang. One of my past relationship ghosts was a rock-'n'-roll singer who had a strong distaste for musical theater. He heard me singing to myself one day (as I would to make myself happy) and stopped me in my tracks saying, "Why do you use that horrible vibrato in your voice? It sounds like wobbly crap. You should cut that out if you ever want to sing well."

Ouch.

Needless to say, I stopped singing to myself when he was around and found myself doing it less and less even when he wasn't present. To this day–years later, I still have moments when I wonder if I should back off of the vibrato as I sing along in the car. That's right–that one crappy moment in time still affects me. It wasn't until I stopped chewing on this depressing story that I heard my voice again and began to break the spell. I decided to share my dormant gift with my husband on our wedding day as a surprise and made the entire wedding party cry (because it was beautiful, not because it hurt their ears–swear).

On the other hand, someone saying something beautiful can fill you for a lifetime. A different ex (more of an angel) was a lover of music, especially of good seventies rock. I was in his friend's room singing along to Stevie Nicks as he played the piano. My ex casually dropped in and listened without us knowing he was there. He applauded afterward, came up, and hugged me, saying he absolutely loved it when I sang and that he wished I would do it more. To this day, I still remember that moment and blush. Moments like that help to exorcise the demons that came before. The point is, we must be so careful with words to help prevent unnecessary baggage.

Stop for a moment and close your eyes (obviously after you've read this). I want you to think about one statement in the past that still hurts you. Something someone said that was so hurtful, it affected the way you saw yourself. What was it in that moment that was so painful and has made it so hard to let go of?

Now think of a moment in time when someone said something so beautiful to you that it makes you smile immediately. Maybe even blush. How has this past comment affected your confidence and life?

Take Aim

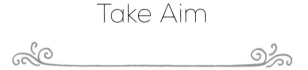

You are officially in pursuit of finding what makes you come alive. You're learning what your amazing qualities and talents are so you can share them with the people around you. You've turned on your "shine" button, and there's a vision of what you would do if there was no chance of failure, because you're in tune with what you're passionate about. Now you can use that passion to wake up your purpose and share your amazing talents with the world. Any residual heartache or past life pain is being ushered away to pave a path for you to take the second step in aiming true—your commitment.

Everything we've done so far is called *setting your intention*. By simply reading this book, you have set the intention to learn and grow. Intention is powerful, but doesn't mean anything if you can't stay focused on your target. Record your answers to the questions in "Aim libs" (page 14) in order to turn your intentions into a focused manifesto of how you want to live your life.

I aimlibs

What does it mean for me to aim true: _____

What are my amazing talents and abilities: _____

What am I passionate about: _____

What is one thing/person/experience I can't let go of that's holding
me back: _____

_____

What am I afraid of: _____

_____

ONCE YOU HAVE ALL OF THESE WRITTEN DOWN AS NOTES,
COMPILE THEM INTO A NOTE WRITTEN TO YOURSELF.
IT WILL GO LIKE THIS:

Aiming true means _____. I will use my ability and talents of
_____ to get out into the world and light my fire and inspire
others to do the same. I am so incredibly passionate about _____
_____ and I will no longer let _____ hold me back or my
fear of _____ stand in my way. I will use my ability to aim
true in every thought and action that I make in order to improve my
life and the conditions around me.

Keep the letter you compose in an important place, and as with
your journal (page 9) I recommend rereading it every month as a constant reminder to keep your aim true, especially when you feel yourself wavering.

Self-Love Prescription

It's important to remind yourself daily of how powerful you are, how incredibly vibrant and gorgeous you already are. In order to not only embrace this but *believe* this, you have to start at the beginning. As soon as you wake up, where's the first place you go? The coffee machine? Headfirst into your cereal bowl? Let's get more primal than that. That's right—the bathroom.

We sleepily pad our way into the bathroom, where we're confronted with a reflection of a not-quite-awake self, and unless you are an actual god or goddess, odds are you may not look your hottest. We take that look in the mirror—lean in close, do a few critical inspections of the tousled hair that no comb can tame, the puffy eyes that will take clinical-strength eye cream to relax, and breath that could make a small dog faint. That's right, as comical as it may seem, we start our day by judging ourselves negatively. Not exactly conducive to an empowered rest of your day.

So how do we combat this? A daily dose of self-love is just what the mind and body need. My dear friend Ash Cebulka may be known as a life coach, but I call her the queen of positive affirmations. When I told her about my quest to figure out what *aim true* means, she recommended a daily dose of positivity to get me on track. She suggested writing a positive affirmation on my bathroom mirror with a Sharpie. This affirmation can be whatever you need it to be—reminding yourself of the good work you're already doing or something that you're working toward. Seeing this message on your bathroom mirror every day is a visual reminder of your intention. So step on up, the doc is in! Get your love prescription right here! Just as eye candy provides a visual feast, heart candy feeds the soul. I've sprinkled Heart Candy exercises throughout the book as sweet reminders and tips to constantly bring you back to a self-loving state.

Sharpie Time!

Writing yourself a self-love prescription is as easy as 1, 2, 3!

1. Rummage through your drawers or hit the local drugstore for a glass-safe Magic Marker.
2. Waltz your way into your bathroom.
3. Write your intention on the bathroom mirror. Write a positive affirmation you're working on in your life. This can be anything: *Aim true. I am not defined by my body. Stop worrying, start living.* Make it your own.

Want to switch up your intention? The marker will come off with a bit of elbow grease, and if necessary, some nail polish remover.

I always have *aim true* written on my bathroom mirror, because it is a daily affirmation for me and how I live my life. Years back, when I was living in Los Angeles, I had more intense affirmations to deal with. I was finishing up year seven in L.A., the city of perfect, pretty, skinny people. While I have many amazing memories of that city, being in the health industry, it felt even more intense and cutthroat, and I suffered from body image issues. I had reached a point where I was being incredibly harsh on myself and found endless areas of my body to critique. I'd stand in front of my bathroom mirror in profile, sticking my stomach out, then sucking it in (aka "bad-good belly dance"), I'd grab handfuls of flesh and make my belly "talk"–the list goes on. It's embarrassing to admit, but it's where I was emotionally. Beneath this ridiculous and demeaning mirror act I'd do with myself, I hated myself for hating myself, which became a descending spiral of habitual negative thought patterns. I knew deep down I didn't want to feel this way, and reminded myself that I was the only one in charge of my own happiness. I decided to take action and get the black Sharpie out (I meant business), and wrote on my mirror *You are PERFECT. You are BEAUTIFUL. You are NOT YOUR BODY.*

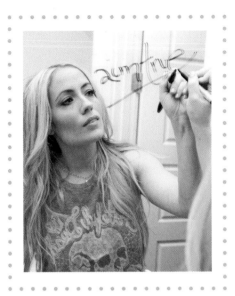

Will writing magic words on your mirror miraculously cleanse you of any negative thoughts you have about yourself? No—but here's the beautiful part. It holds you accountable. You look at your reflection in the mirror, armed with the typical shower of negative thoughts, and then come face-to-face with your affirmation before you can rattle any off. It's that split second where your mind pauses and your eyes connect with a message that your heart has been starving for. That split moment is the space in between, where potential for growth happens. Bear in mind, this won't happen immediately, but it has to start somewhere, and the beginning of your day is a fantastic place to plant the seed.

I See You

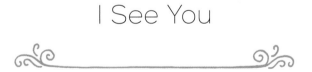

A strong body comes in all different shapes, forms, colors, and sizes. I know this, as I teach and see thousands of different body types, all capable of amazing and strong postures and transitions. Most people struggle with some aspect of their body image—whether they openly admit it or not. I've struggled myself on and off for years, and have learned so much through the highs and lows. I'm a yoga teacher living in the midst of the health world, who doesn't possess the typical "yoga body." I'm not tall, long, and lean. I'm five foot two, incredibly driven and strong, and possess a body that isn't prone to getting super lean.

I've always been praised for my "normal" body. In fact, my first big photo spread in a mainstream magazine was given to me because of that. The photo shoot was focusing on several challenging arm balances, which I happened to be particularly good at. These yoga postures required ample strength, and they loved the fact that I could do these postures with a smile on my face. A compliment is a compliment, and I'll always accept one with a receptive "thank you," but what is a *normal* body, anyway? I was twenty-four at the time; I practiced yoga for two hours a day and ate incredibly clean—I can't say that's the most normal of lifestyles, yet it was mine at the time. People kept commenting on how normal and *real* I was. I said my thank-yous, but thought, *Wow. Good thing I work out as much as I do, and eat as well as I do, or my "normal" body would be a train wreck.*

Flash forward to my thirties: I don't have the luxury to practice daily for two hours, and still eat clean but have learned how to find a good balance in life. My current popular compliment is "You're so brave! I love that you're the curvy girl in yoga! It's so great to see a person who clearly likes to eat! Wow, I love that you're okay with showing your belly."

Brave? I thought brave people battled monsters, not posed to be photographed having fun in a bikini.

It can feel virtually impossible to peacefully exist when the world is constantly throwing out labels—curvy, skinny, slender, athletic, round, normal, etc. Some people are praised for being thin, then called anorexic the next moment, while others are being celebrated as "real," then critiqued for being too big. People love to judge, and there's an unfortunate power in labeling another person, as it seems to take some of the pressure off the person delivering the slam. "If I can find flaws in you, it alleviates the flaws in me." It might make someone temporarily feel better to pick out what's "wrong" with someone else (think gossip magazines and all the fashion faux pas), but ultimately it's a way of deflecting pain instead of dealing with your real emotions about yourself.

So what can we do? Start simple and stop labeling each other. Things like pant size, hair color, and body type hold no weight over the bigger picture. Drop the judgments and see people for their character and energy they give off into the world. Challenge yourself to let up on the judging of others so you can get to what really matters–learning to accept and love yourself as you are.

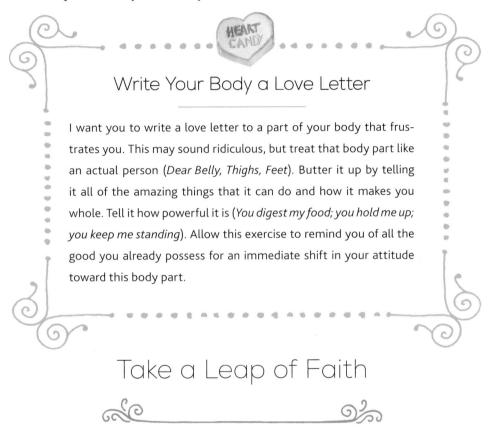

Write Your Body a Love Letter

I want you to write a love letter to a part of your body that frustrates you. This may sound ridiculous, but treat that body part like an actual person (*Dear Belly, Thighs, Feet*). Butter it up by telling it all of the amazing things that it can do and how it makes you whole. Tell it how powerful it is (*You digest my food; you hold me up; you keep me standing*). Allow this exercise to remind you of all the good you already possess for an immediate shift in your attitude toward this body part.

Take a Leap of Faith

When we take away the fear of the unknown, we can release what holds us back and open ourselves up to possibility and whatever may come. I learned this in a very dramatic manner. This is the story of how I broke free from making choices based in fear and decided to show up and shine.

It all started when I was scrolling through Facebook aimlessly and stumbled upon a video of a student of mine making a tandem skydive. This student wasn't exactly the extreme-sport type, yet there she was, getting ready to jump out of a plane. The video followed her preparation, the ascent of the plane, and the terrifying moment of her sitting in the door of the plane. As she exited the plane, her face shone like the sun. She had cleverly written *Shine Bright* in black marker on her palms, which she waved happily at the cameraman as every piece of skin on her face rippled with glee (and 125-mile-per-hour winds). It all accumulated upon her landing into the biggest, most carefree smile I had ever seen.

I was mesmerized. Oh, and sobbing. I didn't know what had come over me. I had never given skydiving a thought until that moment, and suddenly I was calling her up saying, "Hey, I just watched your skydiving video, and I found myself bawling like a baby. So, um, yeah . . . I think I need to jump out of a plane."

She agreed wholeheartedly, and next thing I knew, we'd agreed to jump together the next time we were in the same state—which was about five months away. My heart had officially gone from full-on flutter to slamming into the bottom of my boots.

I had just committed to jumping out of a plane.

I proceeded to ask every person I met from that day on if they had gone skydiving. "Would you do it again?" "Did you like it?" "Did it hurt?" "Did you lose your stomach?" "How was the landing?" Did any of their answers settle my mind? Not even close.

About a month out, I got a phone call from my friend telling me she wasn't going to be able to make it. My immediate reaction? Happy dance. I didn't have to throw myself out of a plane! Unfortunately, I had one more person to call because we had accumulated a third-party jumper. I called him to share the news and waited with bated breath for his reaction. He had already booked the jumps and thought we should keep the reservation regardless, because he was excited to do it.

Damn.

I swallowed my pride and agreed. I used to view these moments as fate or omens, but now realize it's just the universe throwing you a curveball. You put your intention of how you want to aim true out into the world, and the universe doesn't always make it easy for you. In fact, it often likes to test you to see how you react. *Is this what you really want? Here's an out if you're not ready to move past your fear.* I had my freak-out moment, acknowledged it, and kept moving forward with my intention. I was still going to jump out of a plane.

Fast-forward to the fated day. Not a cloud in the sky and blue for miles. I wasn't getting out of this. I arrived at the drop zone, met my fellow jumper, filled out mounds of paperwork, and sat in a room awaiting our tandem masters. The teacher walked in, and he was big—I mean Spartan-warrior big—and I was thrilled. Big, strong man started to give me the lowdown on how everything was going to work, from the gear to the plane ride. My mind started to calm down, because he made it sound simple and actually fun. Meanwhile, my heart continued to betray me and pound as if it wanted permanently out of my body.

The time had come, and we made our way to the plane. We were jumping out of a Skyvan, which is similar to a cargo plane where there's enough space to stand up. We all piled in and took our seats on the floor of the plane as it began to climb. When we got to about five thousand feet, the plane started to level out. I wasn't even strapped to my guy at this point, and started looking around wildly to see what was happening. The next thing I knew, the butt of the plane was open, and one guy stood up. He turned around facing our group, threw us the peace sign, and *whoosh*. He was gone. Just like that.

The butt of the plane closed, and we continued to climb. Evidently we still had higher to go before our jump, which gave me just enough time to contemplate a full-blown panic attack. Every cell in my body was freaking out as my yoga teacher brain took over and calmly reminded me to breathe. *Just breathe. Remember everything your instructor told you. This is going to be amazing!*

I continued to ramble reassuring thoughts to myself until, suddenly, our time arrived. My instructor asked me to sit on his lap so he could snap and tie us together. Once every strap was in its proper place, he told me, "Okay, we need to stand up now. When we stand up, your feet won't be able to touch the ground, so I'm going to need you to bend your knees and tuck your feet in between my legs."

Up we went. I balled myself up into a tiny piece of carry-on. This six-foot-four-inch beast started to march me toward the edge of the plane, while I must have looked like a cross between a rabid koala and a BabyBjörn. We stood on the edge of the plane and had a moment to look out into—well, nothing. This wasn't like standing on the edge of a tall building and experiencing vertigo. This was peering out into the vast unknown, the great wide open of nada. My brain couldn't even begin to comprehend what was going on. He was pointing out to where we were going to jump, and my only mental response was, "Where?! There's absolutely nothing to jump into!"

Just when I couldn't handle this daunting view anymore, he gently pulled my head back and gave me a three count. Out-in-OUT!

We hit the air.

I was legitimately moments away from wetting my pants. I went from the most terrified I'd ever been in my entire life to the most exhilarated in a matter of seconds. It was completely unreal and impossible to explain. It was as if every fear had been eradicated from my mind, and my heart and thoughts were completely fearless and free. The videographer swooped in, threw me the shaka sign, grabbed my hand, spun me around—I was having a ball. You couldn't have wiped that huge open mouthed grin off me if you'd tried. Not even 125-mile-per-hour air blowing into my mouth could stop my joy. I was forever changed.

Standing on the edge of that plane had made everything so clear. What was I so scared of? Yes, skydiving is an extreme sport, but people did this regularly, we were at one of the best drop zones in the world, and I had a pretty strong inkling that my instructor, who did this every day of his life, valued his life just as much as I did mine. So was I afraid I might die? I can't pretend it didn't cross my mind, but I was pretty sure the chances were slim. So, if I wasn't afraid of dying, what was it?

After the jump, it struck me like a ton of bricks—I was terrified of the unknown. Standing on the edge of that plane was so dreadful because

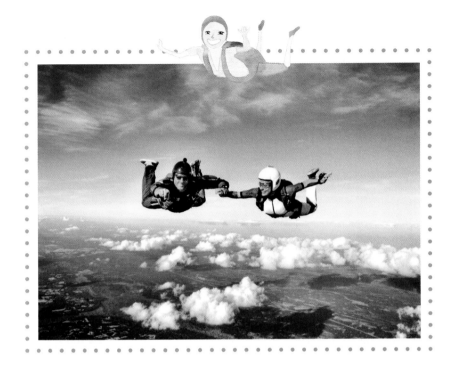

I had no idea what the jump was going to be like. Sure, I'd asked tons of people if they had jumped, if they had liked it. My instructor painted a very clear photo of how fantastic the jump was going to be, but the problem—I didn't know *for sure.* I had to give my complete trust to the unknown, and that absolutely terrified me.

The unknown had always been a scary place to me, a place where uncertainty ruled: *Will I succeed? Will this relationship work out? Will I find happiness if I leave this job for another?*

My first skydive helped me to realize that the unknown isn't terrifying, but rather a place of limitless potential. I realized I had been living a fearful life because I was so frightened by the unknown. From that moment on, I started to look at the choices I had made prior to this day that were ruled by fear. All the things I had done (or not done), because I feared failure or pain. I made a commitment to myself that day to never choose fear again. I would view the unknown as my creative friend full of opportunity. I would remind myself that when I choose fear, I am *not* choosing love, and that is never how I'd want to live.

I had to forget the story—that story we all tell ourselves. The story that allows us to make fearful choices without feeling guilty. The "I can't do that because I don't have enough money" or "I'm not terribly happy in my relationship, but he's good to me and I don't want to start all over" or "I'm not strong enough to become good at this, so I might as well stop now." Little white lies to comfort ourselves. We hardly scratch the surface of a situation, because we're unsure of what may lie beneath.

Uncomfortable or undesirable circumstances can be guides, helping us to realize we're exactly where we should be. Letting go of the story that holds us back frees us up to aim true. The only person standing in your way is the scared storyteller who fears a plot twist. Let go of your fears and take a leap of faith. When you take that leap, keep an eye out for all the opportunities surrounding you.

Oh, and on a side note—that leap of faith resulted in a huge heaping of love. That tandem instructor is now my husband and I'm a certified skydiver with 150 jumps. Just an extra push to let you know the magic happens when we step outside our comfort zone.

Give Your Emotions the Right to Live

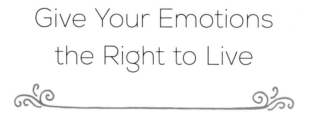

The only person who can make you happy and change your negative habits is *you*. The sooner you can embrace your strength and realize there's no one to blame, the stronger you become. Will there always be holes in the road? Yes, always. Problems are just as prevalent as solutions, but they're also some of our most informative teachers. We need the valleys to create peaks. You might have to fall and climb out of the same hole way more than you'd like to admit. The lesson will be continuously taught until you digest it. So what do we do if we seem to be at the bottom of a bottomless pit of despair?

Give your emotions the right to live.

We all have lessons to learn, and not always the easy way. When you're at the bottom of that stupid hole and can't find your way out—you're going to get angry! You'll experience negative thoughts and ample doses of judgment. You can't conquer these emotions by ignoring them. When these emotions linger unaddressed, they make us feel shame. Next thing you know, you're upset for being upset and entering a downward spiral of negativity.

The teachings of yoga instruct us to lose judgment and reactivity. The goal is to enter a state of peace where we can observe without rash reaction and accept people and situations for exactly as they are. Connecting with and voicing your emotions without judgment is a key to loving who you are right now.

Compare your emotional needs to the breakdown of a toddler. Think the terrible twos—that phase in life when children have so much they want to say without the tools to properly express themselves. This lack of expression turns into full-blown rage and frustration. The meltdown comes from being unable to speak and share their emotions. If parents discipline a child for this behavior, it only makes it worse. They're saying it isn't all right to have those natural feelings of frustration, and that they don't understand or empathize with the situation.

Like the toddler's tantrum, pushing emotions down or ignoring them only worsens matters. But what if we attempt to understand these feelings and accept them in their current state? Start interacting with your inner child when it comes to your emotions. It's okay to feel! Allow yourself to voice your emotions without judgment. This emotional freedom and unedited honesty allows us to embrace happiness. We can move through natural reactions, allow real emotions to flow that need release, and then feel clear and exorcised of the demons that shame us for feeling the way we do. You are right, you are perfect, you are exactly where you need to be.

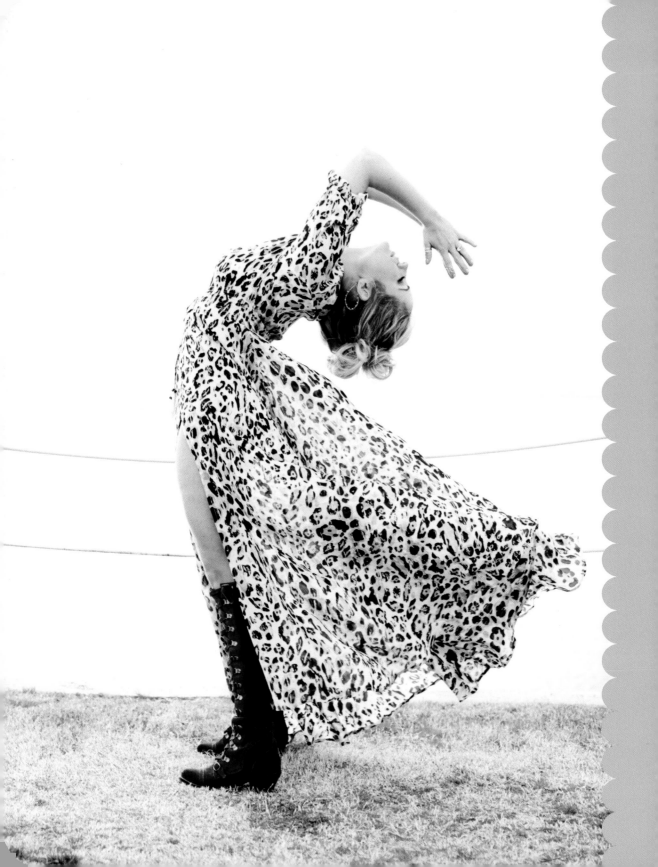

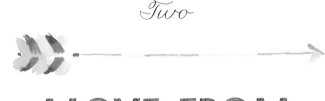

Two

MOVE FROM *the* INSIDE OUT

You have an amazing, capable, and gorgeous body. Is loving yourself all you need to do in order to get the most kick-ass physique in the world? Yes and no. Just being happy isn't going to make your physical body magically shift into a god or goddess form. You will need to put the physical work in to complement the emotional, but here's the cool part—when you love yourself, the physical aspect doesn't feel nearly as important. When we aim true with our physical bodies, we're defined by how we feel, which allows energy to radiate.

We can embrace happiness and choose to be our own personal cheerleader if we desire happiness. We just need to remember that we're on the same team as our body. It can't support us without our support—physical, mental, and emotional.

I'm confident that the body and all its parts actually have feelings, and if we bash them enough, it will rebel. Talk enough trash about your legs, and they'll stop supporting you. Unhappy with your arms, and they'll hang limp at your sides instead of embracing loved ones. Rather than hating on the only body we get, lift it up with positive reinforcement and watch your confidence grow. This is your body, and it was given to you in its form for a reason. Trust that and rock it.

My Belly-Bashing Aha Moment

The best thing we can do to help ourselves and others is to speak clear, positive, powerful statements about ourselves. Let me paint you a picture.

I lead yoga retreats a few times a year and once chose Mexico for a New Year's Eve retreat. Yes, I'm the genius who thought it would be a good idea to romp around in a bikini after a full holiday month of indulgences and celebration. Day one of our retreat, and everyone was already hitting up the hot tub, so I rummaged through my bathing suits to find one that had an extra fringy top that dangled down over my midsection. I tied it on and joined the human soup bowl to socialize with my students. One student, Holly, was a beautiful girl who had struggled with eating disorders for years. She was still rather frail, but was taking each day at a time to empower herself. I was rambling on with my students as the "can't believe we have to be in bathing suits" topic inevitably came up. I joked that I loved my bathing suit because the fringe hung so low it covered up my bloated holiday belly. Holly stopped in her tracks and gaped at me. She immediately replied, "How could you ever say something like that about your body? You have an amazing, beautiful body. Don't ever say something like that."

I will never forget the expression of disappointment and hurt in her face when I jokingly (but ultimately negatively) bashed my body. It made me realize how socially acceptable it is. How often does someone pay you a compliment where you simply reply "Thank you" as opposed to "Oh, this old thing?" or "Are you kidding me? I look like a cow." We use humor as a way to deflect what we really feel—pain and insecurity. I had let my insecurity come out in the form of a joke, when all I was doing was giving everyone in that hot tub permission to do the same. I was their teacher—the person they looked up to, the woman who gave them the tools to succeed—and there I was glorifying self-deprecating humor.

Speaking ill of yourself will do nothing but hurt you and give those listening to you permission to say the same about themselves. I've wasted time thinking I'm too short and curvy to be an inspiring fitness figure, but the truth is—this is my body! I've never rocked six-pack abs, and even at my strongest, I still have a "soft" look, yet my body has been so good to me. It responds to good food and physical care. It can perform difficult poses or workouts with the most Spartan of body types. Each of us comes with our own talents and our own internal struggles.

When you empower yourself to accept compliments, to openly speak positive statements about your body, and to appreciate your talents, you encourage others to follow suit. Thoughts are like magic and words are like spells. Be careful with what you cast. Practice white magic—openly embrace your body. Thinking positive thoughts about your body leads to speaking them out loud. Once these spells are cast, they become a reality, but it all starts with finding the right ingredients to brew the perfect potion.

DELETE HAPPY

Ever take an amazing image of yourself only to realize you didn't like the way it looked? Maybe it wasn't flattering to your belly, or the angle brought out your insecurities, but meanwhile the overall image is amazing! It either immediately gets deleted or dies in the archives of your phone. I dare you to post these images! Drop the need to be filtered. If the energy of the image inspires you, it will do the same for others. The world needs more people being raw and honest. Step into that power and own your beauty!

I posted the photo on page 30 on the eve of my thirty-second birthday with an accompanying photo of me on the beach showing my cellulite. It was perhaps the most popular post I've ever shared, and I still get letters thanking me for being open and honest about the reality we all deal with but try to cover up with a mask of perfection. Let's start a revolution of radical acceptance and love by keeping it real!

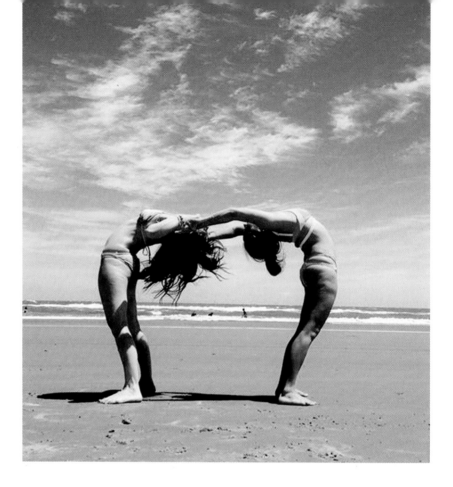

Body Renaissance

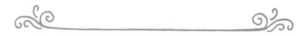

This is the only body you're going to get on this go-around. It may sound crass, but I view my body simply—as a meat suit. It's a vehicle that I've been given to steer me around this life as I fill it up with amazing (and occasionally horrible yet educational) decisions. This meat suit allows me to get from point A to point B, to embrace the ones I love, to lift those up who need help, to prepare food to nourish myself, and to constantly prove that I'm pure magic when I apply myself with patience. This suit is constantly changing. Sometimes it will be strong and unstoppable. Other times it will be soft, gentle, and subdued. Occasionally, it will feel

Aim True

broken and painful. Eventually it will die—and this isn't a bad thing; it's simply the circle of life. This vehicle is meant to last for only so long, so we do our best in caring for it on a daily basis.

Judging it and labeling it will only make it disintegrate faster. Don't give your beauty an expiration date. Age will alter our bodies, but it doesn't mean we give in to the clock and throw in the towel. Everyone told me that once you turn thirty your body will completely change (and not in a good way). Then I've heard nothing gets easier after forty, and the comments continue, pertaining to each decade. It saddens me that milestone birthdays are seen as new limitations of our body's ability to be strong and beautiful, when each birthday should be a celebration of our knowledge and how beautiful our life experiences make us. It's crucial that we take care of our health physically, with the way we eat and exercise, and that we care for ourselves emotionally as well. This emotional support system is often much stronger than our physical capabilities, and it can be the extra kick in the pants we need to get off our butts into a physical activity. When we emotionally love ourselves, we *want* to be the best versions of ourselves.

Does that mean if we emotionally love ourselves we can throw caution to the wind and dance in a rainstorm of potato chips? Just being happy isn't going to make you physically healthy, but here's the cool part—when you love yourself, the physical aspect isn't nearly as important to you. It isn't easy to drop years of preconceived notions of what we look like and how that defines us. All I ask is that you try. Your meat suit is lovely, my dear. Let's start using it to its full abilities.

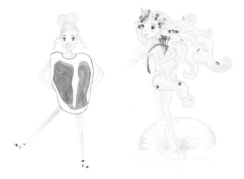

Work Your Body

We're figuring out how to love the skin we're in, but we also need to get ready to *work* the skin we're in. A physical routine will not only be the perfect buddy system to your emotional one, but it will inspire you, release endorphins, and give you a strong connection to routine.

While teaching workshops around the world has allowed me to see amazing beauty in all different corners of the world, this type of schedule is not conducive to any semblance of routine. I often live off airport/plane food and find myself constantly struggling to stay active and hydrated. This kind of lifestyle has taken a major toll on my physical body, because I lack the routine of nutritional and physical outlets that I maintain when I'm home. I ultimately made a concerted effort to chop my travel schedule in half to support my health. If you fall into the category where finding a regular schedule or finding the time seems impossible because of your life, try your best. For me, it meant waking up earlier to do ten minutes of yoga or to sit and meditate before I started my day. It means packing protein powders, probiotics, and healthy snacks in case my options were limited on the road. It meant packing my big reusable water bottle and filling it regularly to keep myself hydrated and my digestive system happy whatever the change of scenery. You *can* work your body regardless of whatever environmental or time constraints you're under.

It's time to create a routine. Your body wants to be used to its full potential, so give it a chance! Carve out at least fifteen minutes from your day and dedicate that time to your physical body. It can be taking a walk outside, doing a yoga practice, going for a run, lifting weights, or popping in your favorite workout DVD. Some of us are such creatures of habit that we want the same sequence and workout daily—great! Whatever works for you! I tend to fall into the "easily bored" category, so my routine consists of mixing up yoga, running, jujitsu, sparring, long dog walks, and outdoor activities. I try to do something different each day to keep my mind stimulated, but what's most important is to *do something every day*. Try to break a sweat daily. Try something that challenges you without breaking your spirit. Find activities that are stimulating, creative, and fun (yoga and martial arts are two of my favorites) so that you look forward to your physical time slot.

Will there come days where an hour of sweating is impossible? Yes! It's life! Do what you can, and when you get that moment to physically connect, give yourself to it completely. Don't be attached to duration or calorie count—just commit to doing something. It's not always easy in the beginning, but once you fall into the routine, you'll crave it just as much as you would a piece of chocolate.

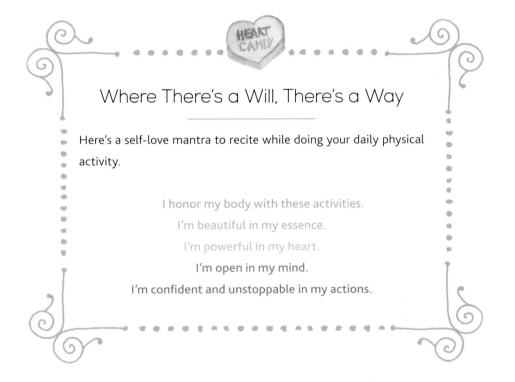

Where There's a Will, There's a Way

Here's a self-love mantra to recite while doing your daily physical activity.

I honor my body with these activities.
I'm beautiful in my essence.
I'm powerful in my heart.
I'm open in my mind.
I'm confident and unstoppable in my actions.

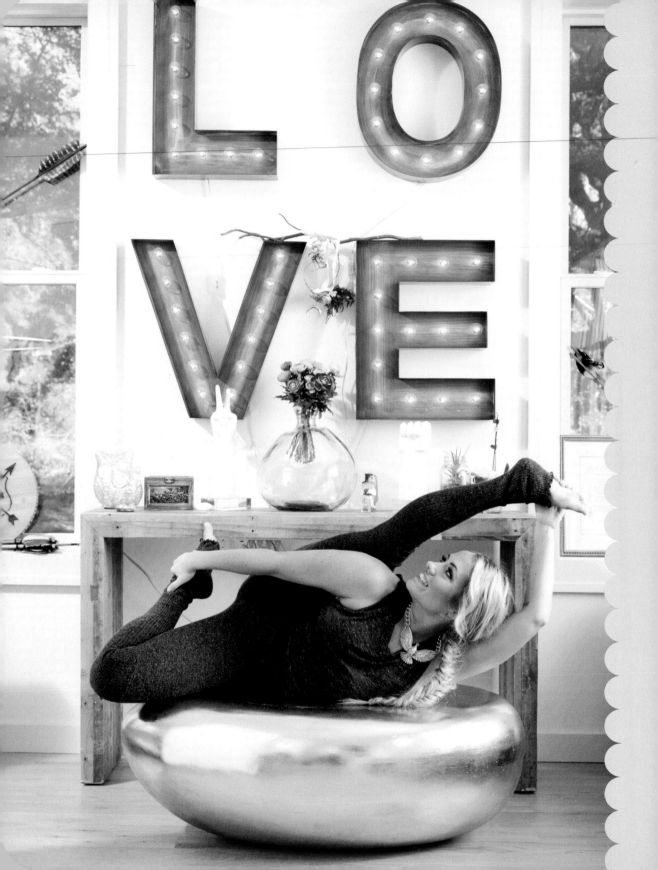

Three

GET ON THE MAT

Yoga falls into a unique category, in the sense that it can be called a workout, a lifestyle, and even a spiritual path. Yoga asana (the actual postures) and philosophy go back a good five thousand years. Anything that can survive that long has some serious staying power, as well as a beautiful ability to adapt.

I've been incredibly blessed to teach this amazing craft for over ten years watching the light turn on behind thousands of eager eyes. Yoga is nothing short of magic. I compare teaching yoga to blowing empowering pixie dust into people's hearts and minds. People are completely transformed by this practice.

It starts with curiosity—maybe someone wants to get in shape or lose some weight. Maybe they've heard about how popular this "yoga" thing is, or it just so happens that their gym offers a class and it fits their schedule. These casual first encounters normally lead to an enticing courtship that evolves into a full-blown life commitment.

Yoga affects the way people think, move, eat, and interact. Everyone comes in with a set of limiting beliefs about what their body is capable of achieving. With mindful application of theory, dedication to the practice, and a big dose of support from the teacher, they succeed. Postures or movements that they never dreamed possible are suddenly a common affair. Their toes, once foreign, are now touchable, part of the same zip code as their fingertips.

Balancing on their hands becomes almost as common as standing firmly on two feet. What was considered impossible becomes an anticipated challenge to try something new.

The Body as the Bow

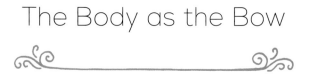

The goal of yoga isn't to be a trained dolphin, it's to be fully in tune with your vehicle and use it to its optimal ability. Yoga allows us to learn how to aim true in our physical bodies. Imagine your body as the bow and your intention and talents as the arrow. Your body is always the safe hearth to your passions. It is also constantly changing. Sometimes it will perform at its peak ability, while other days, you won't be entirely sure if you're in the right body at all. Aim true yoga means we're open to whatever shows up on the mat, because we possess the ability to alter our mind-set and practice to adapt to whatever condition we're in. All this possibility falls into our lap when we apply our aim true philosophy:

Show up with strong intention. I want to succeed. I'm open to falling and getting back up. No isn't part of my vocabulary. I love myself exactly as I am and have every tool I need to succeed. My will is stronger than fate.

This attitude prevents us from dwelling in the pits of frustration over the body's abilities. Will we always nail a pose? No. Does that mean it's okay to screw up? You better believe it! Chill out, young Jedi. You've got plenty of time to rule the world or—for starters—all four corners of your yoga mat. You'll only be a beginner once, so enjoy!

There's something so thrilling about the start of something new. It challenges the mind, makes us show up fully and honestly. Whether you are completely new to yoga, trying aim true yoga for the first time, or reengaging with this practice, remember to embrace your beginner mentality as you tackle your practice, because it's exactly that—a practice. We're not trying to master yoga, to conquer it, or even complete it. We're inviting it into our lives, asking if it'd like to hold our hand forever, so don't rush the courtship. It's incredibly fun.

Ride the Waves

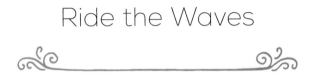

The story of Artemis is a perfect example of what it means to be yourself. It wasn't until I felt the societal pressures myself as a young woman in the world that I could truly respect and understand Artemis's empowerment in riding against the tide. This woman knew exactly what she wanted and wasn't afraid to ask for it. She paved the way for aiming true for all of us. It's so important that we remind ourselves that aiming true is not always easy.

Aim true yoga helps us remember that we're exactly who and where we should be in life. The yoga postures won't go easy on us—they'll challenge our strength, flexibility, awareness, and durability. These poses teach us that we must show up as ourselves. Not a version of ourselves that we wish to be or an emulation of someone we are inspired by (though of course role models and teachers can offer guidance and inspiration). Embrace your body and your talents and know that your message—as personal and unique as it may be—is the key to reaching your goals. We shine when we're sharing a message that reflects who we are.

Remember, aiming true is the ability to be yourself both on and off the mat. The yoga mat is a safe place to succeed and fail. Listen to your body, move in the direction that it beckons, and know that taking it down a notch when everything in your being tells you to slow down is often way more powerful than kicking it up. This is where intention becomes key.

Set Your Intention

Setting intention at the beginning of the yoga practice is the same way that we aim true by setting our intention on what makes our heart beat. Many yoga practices start in a pose called Mountain, or *Samasthiti*, which translates to "equal standing," or as my teacher would often say, a state of bliss and joy. You bring your palms together at the heart space into a mudra (gesture) called Anjali, which symbolizes devotion and respect. I always encourage my students to take a moment of pause here before we dive into the physical aspects of the practice. It's a sweet moment, where you can stop before you begin. Now is the time to set your intention and make your aim true. Ponder the following questions to help you create a powerful intention:

Why am I here?

Why am I drawn to this practice?

Why do I love yoga?

How do I feel right now?

How do I want to feel during the practice?

How do I want to feel when I'm done?

Whom would I like to dedicate this practice to?

Remember that intention can be complex—something you've been working on for months or years. It can encompass huge lifetime goals, or it can be something as simple as saying "I want to have fun today. I want to remember to be playful even when the posture is frustrating or challenging," or "I'm in a crap mood, and I'd like to feel better and let go of my baggage," or "I just really want to survive this class. I'm exhausted and know I'll feel better for doing this."

It can be fairly common to set an intention at the beginning of your practice only to completely forget it a mere ten minutes into the class. I constantly remind my students to come back to their original intention and *use* it, because herein lies the problem: yoga is *hard*! It's meant to challenge us and push us outside of our comfort zone. These postures are not always easily attainable, so it's also fairly common to end up feeling defeated. If we can keep the intention strong (e.g., "I want to have fun and see the silver lining in every success even when I flop on my mat"), we truly walk away from the practice stronger and changed. Achieving this kind of attitude is even more challenging than a freestanding handstand. This is the attitude that teaches you how to be unapologetically you on and off the mat—and reap all the benefits.

Be Luminous

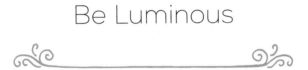

I like to think of asana as the physical manifestation of how we're feeling on the inside. We use these postures as a physical language or a moving prayer. Our ability to set intention infuses the attitude and shape of the pose so we can convey our energy without using words. Don't get caught up on the aesthetics of the posture, but rather drive your intention and energy into every line of your body.

A backbend is one of the most beautiful postures in yoga. It's open, expressive, and beautifully vulnerable. Some students are naturally flexible in this region of the body, while others swear they were born with cement in their upper back and hip flexors. I have a theory about backbends. Imagine you're running from a saber-toothed tiger. You're hoofing it, but to no avail. The beast is almost upon you, so what options do you have left? Drop into a tiny ball, pull your knees to your chest, and wrap yourself around your legs in hopes that you protect your vital organs. When we do a backbend, we are fully exposing every organ, all of ourselves to the world saying, "I totally trust this moment! I believe nothing will attack me and that I am as safe as safe can be. I give in to this pose and moment knowing I am safe, nurtured, and happy."

If you attempt a backbend and fall into more of a tight backbend or one where you feel claustrophobic, it may not be so much of a physical response as it is emotional. It's time to tap in physically *and* emotionally. The backbend will come with a perfect blend of physical discipline and our ability to work through our emotional baggage. Backbends urge us to be content with who we are and to build our strength and confidence. Let these poses be your teachers and open up the doors of possibility. As you find this blend, your pose will indeed be a physical manifestation of your internal intention.

Beyond the physical benefits and symbolism of our core emotions, yoga postures also teach us how to exist and react in real life. If we apply ourselves enough, we can go deeper into a backbend, build the upper body strength to hold a handstand, or flow through a ninety-minute class.

Accept that everything shows up for a reason. Our goal is to stay nonreactive and be observant so we can learn and become stronger. This is the reason we do yoga–to grow. To become a better version of ourselves. To aim true and see the lesson is all that truly matters. All you have to do is show up and do your best.

Comparison Stops Here

Yoga comprises glorious postures meant for all bodies, but let's be totally honest—there are many postures and depths of variations that are meant only for the super flexible or incredibly disciplined (which often translates to stubborn) practitioners. Let's imagine you're in yoga class and you've had a particularly hard day:

You place your mat down and are starting to fill your intention tank with positivity when you hear—*thwaap*—someone settling next to you. You turn to see an Amazonian beauty limberly warming her body up before class. Your head is about as tall as her belly button, and her hair is so shiny it hurts to look directly in her vicinity.

Sigh . . .

Bring your gaze back onto your mat. Keep your intention strong. Doesn't matter that your shirt is inside out and you're pretty sure you haven't washed these leggings in a while. You're not concerned at all being next to the ambassador for Most Gorgeous Yoga Outfits Ever.

You start to practice. You arrive at handstands, which you've been working on for months. In fact, you've had moments of lingering air-time in the middle of the room. The taste of balancing success is right on the tip of your tongue. You start to kick up with hopes of flight time, but as fate will have it, your body isn't game. It's telling you to sit the hell down and take the day off from inverting. You catch an unfortunate glimpse of Wonder Woman in handstand next to you. Her effortless inversion goes on for days as you finally crumple into a melted child's pose.

You have a choice. Are you going to give in to comparison and let someone else's success ruin your practice? Or did you come to yoga to feel good?

One of my favorite quotes that may have come from Eleanor Roosevelt is "Comparison is the thief of joy." You can compare yourself with the people around you until you're blue in the face, and it won't do a single thing except encourage poor self-esteem. Will you always have at least one person in your life who's "better" than you—on the mat, at your job, in your family? Always. Will you get closer to aiming true by dwelling on comparison? You won't even be able to pull your arrow back to take aim.

Stop comparing. Start living. It's up to you to live your life, not others. Comparing yourself with others is like living in permanent la-la land. You control your abilities and actions, so take the reins! If you can get beyond any kind of jealousy that arrives on the mat, you will be a champion for nonreactivity off the mat. You'll be able to see people and situations for what they are, not what you've painted in your head. This is an incredibly powerful tool, but there's one more I want you to wrap your head around:

Stop comparing yourself with yourself.

More than comparing themselves with others, people struggle with self-comparison and critique. I've found this to be my biggest road bump as I grow older in the health industry. I've had the unfortunate privilege to see my body photographed from the ripe age of twenty-one to the present. I can't count the amount of times I've wanted my twentysomething body back, or how much stronger, thinner, able my body was then compared with what I have now. I'll be having a particularly confident day only to run across an old beautiful image that degrades my current views on how I look. Or I'll try to execute a yoga transition that was once seamless and find that I can't even make it start to happen.

This trap of comparing yourself with a younger version is dangerous and unrealistic. You can't be who you were yesterday; you're a new person now! While a younger, suppler body seems alluring, the idea of emotionally reliving my twenties makes my heart quiver. We only get better with age. You're always getting better and nothing is ever too late. My body may not be the same svelte one that I rocked at twenty-four, but my mind and heart are full with experience and stories that trump any body part. Every moment serves its purpose. The previous chapters of your life were fascinating, but remember, they were only setting you up for the adventures of the chapter to come. The best we can do is show up, set our intention to aim true, do our best, and repeat the next day. You'll rest your head on your pillow every night knowing that you did exactly what you could and needed to. This is how we live in the present moment and embrace whatever it offers us.

HEART CANDY

Change Your Thought Patterns

Slay the comparison dragon by changing the way you speak and think. Replace any "I used to" and "I'm not" with I AM.

~~I'm not~~ I AM strong.

~~I used to be~~ I AM flexible.

~~I'm not~~ I AM capable.

~~I'm not~~ I AM brave.

~~I'm not good~~ I AM enough.

~~I'm not where I want to~~ I AM exactly where I should be.

Developing a Yoga Practice

Yoga has changed me in so many ways. Beyond the physical aspects on the mat, it has allowed me to open up my eyes to every situation, good or bad. There's a lesson waiting for you in every conversation, an opportunity to grow in every disagreement, and a chance to strengthen your love with every brave piece of honesty.

Yoga lets me be right here, right now, and I want to offer this gift to you as well. Some of you reading this may be devout practitioners, while some of you may have only heard about it. The beauty of yoga is that it's open to all ages, sizes, genders, races, and levels of ability. The challenge is seeking out the style that suits you best.

I was personally trained in the Yogaworks style, which is a blend of Ashtanga, Iyengar, and Viniyoga (a blend of asana, breathwork, meditation). I've experienced a plethora of styles and practiced Ashtanga for years. My resulting style can be labeled as Vinyasa Flow, but with my own personal spin. I pride myself on making the practice accessible, playful, and exciting while keeping my students educated, aware of alignment, and safe.

Yoga can be practiced safely on a daily basis, but I'm a firm believer in taking at least one day off to rest. A good goal would be three to four times a week. Most public classes are sixty to ninety minutes long. If you are blessed with the time, accessibility, and finances to practice in a class, please do it. Your practice will truly blossom under the guidance of a senior teacher who can physically assist you and keep you safe. A good teacher will make you *want* to practice. My teacher, Maty Ezraty, was so dynamic that I'd even move doctor's appointments to make sure I could get into her room on a daily basis. Her style of teaching spoke to me, lit me up, and made me want to be a better student. Keep exploring until you find a teacher you love.

Practicing online and creating a home practice are two ways to do

Aim True

yoga solo in the comfort of your own home. There's no embarrassment about practicing in front of people, no frustrating commute, no need to get a babysitter. It's also much easier on the wallet. Check out "A Few of My Favorite Things" on page 311 for some of my preferred DVDs and websites.

Developing a home practice takes attention and discipline. I'll often start my home practice only to notice I need to sweep or hear the phone ring or even get distracted by my dog. That being said, it's one of the best things you can do for yourself because that "studio" is open 24/7! Begin your own personal practice with the sequences in the following chapter.

FIND YOUR STYLE

How do you find what style is best for you? Try them all! Start with the one that appeals to your general personality, but explore all venues, as there's something to gain from each approach.

Are you . . .	Then try . . .
Athletic	Ashtanga, Power, or Vinyasa Flow for dynamic movement in connection with breath
Cerebral	Iyengar for its attention to detail
Spiritual	Kundalini for its chants, breathwork, and meditation
Stressball	Yin or Restorative to stretch, relax, and unwind

6 STEPS TO CREATING
A HOME PRACTICE

STEP 1: **Create a sacred space.** This can be a small unused room, a corner of your bedroom, a spot in your living room, or even a place outside on your deck (weather permitting). All you need is a space free from distractions and large enough for you to place your yoga mat and reach your arms wide and overhead.

STEP 2: **Make it cozy!** Light some candles, burn some sage or incense, play music that soothes or motivates you, and put on clothing that makes you feel good. Creating an altar (see next page) also helps to focus your intention and energy.

STEP 3: **Set a date.** Try to practice at the same time every day. Drop what you're doing and remind yourself that this small amount of time will improve the entire rest of your day. Notice how establishing this routine affects your mood and physicality. It's worth it.

STEP 4: **Create a buddy system.** I used to live in central Florida with very little access to yoga, so I had a yoga date at my house with a friend twice a week. We made it sacred and kept each other accountable.

STEP 5: **Commit to completing your practice.** Determine how much time you want to dedicate—five, ten, twenty minutes—and then stay on the mat for that amount of time. Whether you have a sequence to follow or prefer to move in an organic, flowy way, let your practice take over for that set time.

STEP 6: **Don't think—just practice.** Don't pin yourself down to thinking only one style or duration qualifies as a proper practice. There will be days when you are strong like a bull and other days when you'll mew like the runt of the litter. By now you know that one of those days is no better than the others.

CREATE AN ALTAR

We can be connected and spiritual anywhere in the world, but it helps to create a space conducive to appreciation, gratitude, and connection. An altar can be an entire room or a small table with symbolic items on it. Create an altar the way you would decorate a mantel—full of images and symbols that create good feelings and memories. Here are some ideas:

- Symbols of hope and inspiration. (My altar has my childhood teddy bear to remind me to be playful, and a wand that my mother gave me to remind me that magic is real and I can create it.)

- Pictures of your loved ones, teachers, people who inspire you.

- Sculptures/physical representations of deities. (What deities do you relate to? This can be Shiva, the Virgin Mary, or even Artemis.)

- Beautiful, living things (plants, flowers).

- Storage for yoga and spirituality books.

- Something to write with and a sacred journal. (It's also a good place to store important letters or notes.)

- Candles, incense, and holders to help you relax or focus, to be lit and extinguished at the beginning and end of a practice.

- A fireproof bowl in which to burn incense, resin, paper inscribed with things you want to let go of.

- A bundle of dried sage to burn and cleanse the space before your practice. (I'll sage myself to dispel negative energy after a long day around frustrating people or situations.)

- Mala beads (for Japa meditation practice, page 248), to keep them energetically charged.

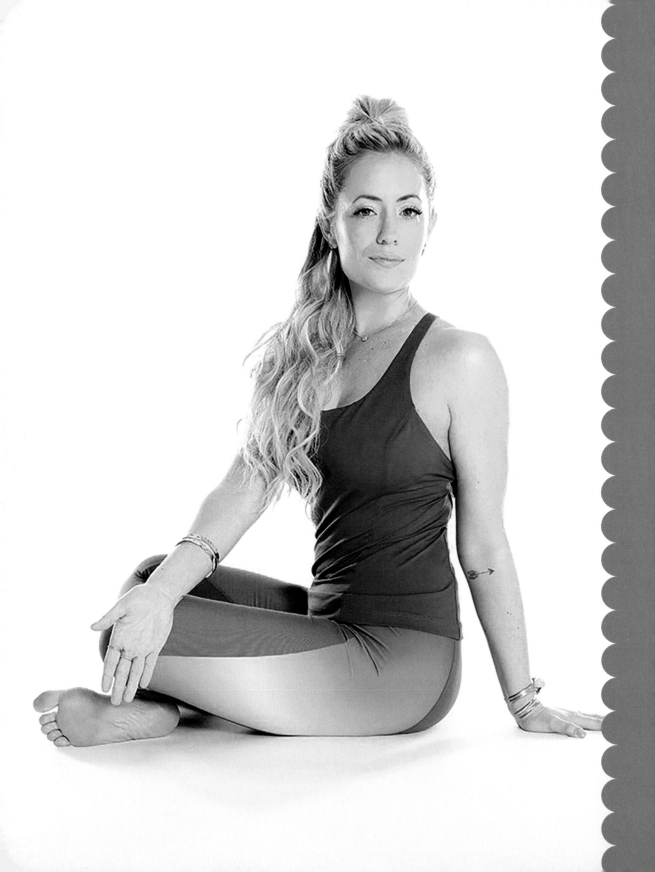

Four

AIM TRUE YOGA: 6 SEQUENCES *to* PUT *into* PRACTICE

Remember those jitters you'd get as a child before the first day of school? These feelings aren't that different from the ones a newbie yogi gets when unrolling a new yoga mat. *Will I fit in? Can I keep up? Am I even made for this whole yoga thing?* To answer all of your questions simply—yes. Anyone and everyone can do yoga; the catch is we need to be willing to adapt to what the body needs instead of what the ego tells us we want.

All you'll need for the sequences in the following chapter is a skidless yoga mat (or yoga towel if it's slippery). I also recommend having two yoga blocks and a strap to help build stability and flexibility, as well as a blanket or bolster to prop you up for meditation.

Sun Salutations
(Surya Namaskara)

I want to start you off with two simple sequences called Sun Salutations A and B. These flows are commonly used at the beginning of yoga classes to build heat and flexibility before entering the main postures. I'll often practice the salutations on their own if I don't have much time, or whenever I need to stretch out and feel good. Think of evoking energy, of starting your day (or restarting at this moment) with powerful intention, and focus on feeling good!

Once you feel confident with Sun Salutation A, you can follow with the B variation. It's virtually the same sequence, but longer, with the addition of Warrior I and Chair to burn extra fire in your legs and hips, and a few extra *Vinyasas* to strengthen your upper body and help flush out your spine.

Sun Salutation A

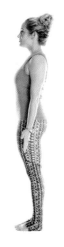

TADASANA
(MOUNTAIN POSE)

Stand tall, with your feet together and your arms by your sides. Gaze forward and take a few deep breaths to focus.

URDHVA HASTASANA
(UPWARD-FACING HANDS)

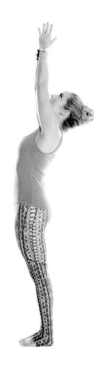

INHALE

Open your arms wide and press your palms together overhead. Keep the base of your neck relaxed, but arms extending long.

UTTANASANA
(STANDING FORWARD BEND)

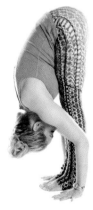

EXHALE

Keep the length in your spine as you hinge from your hips to fold forward. Bring your hands to your shins or palms to the ground. Avoid rounding in your back.

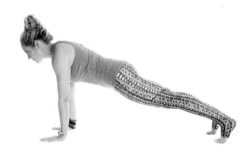

ARDHA UTTANASANA
(HALF STANDING FORWARD BEND)

INHALE

Keep your hands on the ground or shins as you extend your gaze and torso forward. Roll your shoulders back and extend long through your heart.

PLANK INTO *CHATURANGA*
(FOUR-LIMBED STAFF POSE)

EXHALE

Keep your gaze forward as you step back into a pre-push-up. Stack your shoulders over your wrists with straight arms; keep your hips in line with your shoulders and your feet hip width apart.

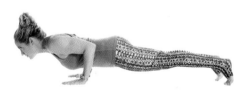

Hold for a full breath or continue on the same exhale to bend your elbows to 90 degrees. Gaze forward, elbows over your wrists, shoulders lowered in line with your elbows. Hug the elbows tight to your ribs and keep your core and legs engaged.

URDHVA MUKHA SVANASANA
(UPWARD-FACING DOG)

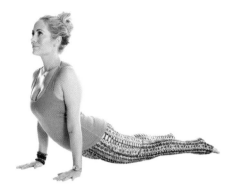

INHALE

Flip onto the toenail side of your feet as you drop your hips and straighten your arms. Relax the base of your neck and gently pull your chest through the gateway of your arms. Gaze forward or slightly up.

ADHO MUKHA SVANASANA
(DOWNWARD-FACING DOG)

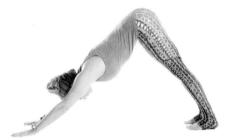

EXHALE

Press the ground away as you lift your hips and roll back onto the soles of your feet. Pull your body back into an inverted V shape with your ears in line with your arms, ribs in, legs active and working toward straight. Hold for 5 full breaths.

Gaze forward at the bottom of your fifth exhale and step or jump to meet your hands.

ARDHA UTTANASANA
(HALF STANDING FORWARD BEND)

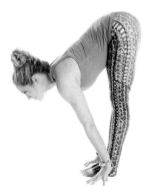

INHALE

Keep your hands down as you extend your torso and gaze forward.

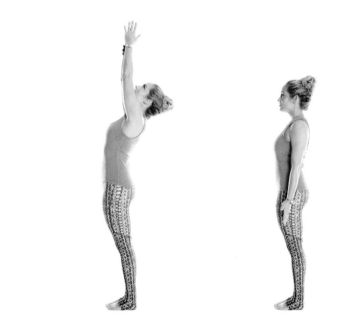

UTTANASANA
(STANDING FORWARD
BEND)

URDHVA HASTASANA
(UPWARD-FACING
HANDS)

TADASANA
(MOUNTAIN POSE)

EXHALE
Maintain the length and
fold long over your legs.

INHALE
Sweep your arms wide
and overhead as you
stand up straight. Gaze
toward your fingertips.

EXHALE
Release your arms to
your sides.

Sun Salutation B

TADASANA
(MOUNTAIN POSE)

Stand tall with your feet together and your
arms by your side. Gaze forward and take
a breath to focus.

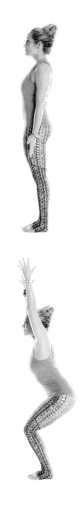

UTKATASANA
(CHAIR POSE)

INHALE
Bend your knees and sink your hips as
you raise your arms straight overhead.
Keep the weight in your heels, shinbones
pressing back, spine long, and gaze forward or up. If you can keep your shoulders
relaxed and arms straight, join your palms
together.

UTTANASANA
(STANDING FORWARD BEND)

EXHALE
Keep the length in your spine as you
hinge from your hips and straighten your
legs to fold forward. Bring your hands to
your shins or palms to the ground. Avoid
rounding in your back.

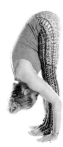

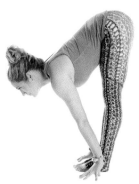

INHALE

Keep your hands on the ground or shins as you extend your gaze and torso forward. Roll your shoulders back and extend long through your heart.

PLANK INTO *CHATURANGA*
(FOUR-LIMBED STAFF POSE)

EXHALE

Keep your gaze forward as you step back into a pre-push-up. Stack your shoulders over your wrists with straight arms, keep your hips in line with your shoulders and your feet hip width apart.

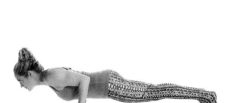

Hold for a full breath or continue on the same exhale to bend your elbows to 90 degrees. Gaze forward, elbows over your wrists, shoulders lowered in line with your elbows. Hug the elbows tight to your ribs and keep your core and legs engaged.

URDHVA MUKHA SVANASANA
(UPWARD-FACING DOG)

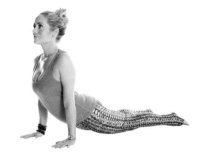

INHALE

Flip onto the toenail side of your feet as you drop your hips and straighten your arms. Relax the base of the neck and gently pull your chest through the gateway of your arms. Gaze forward or slightly up.

ADHO MUKHA SVANASANA
(DOWNWARD-FACING DOG)

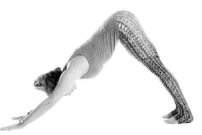

EXHALE

Press the ground away as you lift your hips and roll back onto the soles of your feet. Pull your body back into an inverted V shape with your ears in line with your arms, ribs in, legs active and working toward straight.

VIRABHADRASANA I (WARRIOR I)

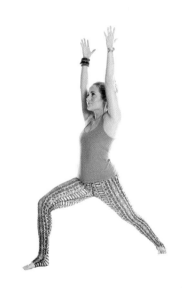

INHALE

Step your right foot forward to meet your right thumb and spin your back foot flat so that you have heel-to-heel alignment. Keep your front knee bent as you lift your torso and arms straight up. Square your ribs and hips forward as you continue to root into the outer edge of your back foot. Reach your arms shoulder width apart or draw the palms to touch.

VINYASA

Vinyasa (Plank to *Chaturanga* to Upward-Facing Dog to Downward-Facing Dog) is the core action in Sun Salutations. It creates a lovely flow that transitions you in between sides of your body. Refer to these pages whenever *Vinyasa* is mentioned in sequences. You'll normally step back into Plank from a standing pose and continue the sequence from there.

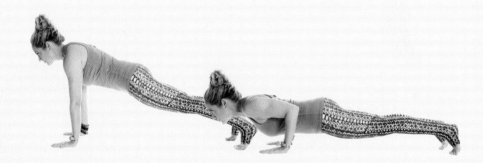

Plank:

Inhale, keep your gaze forward as you step back into a pre-push-up. Stack your shoulders over your wrists with straight arms; keep your hips in line with your shoulders and feet hip width apart.

Chaturanga:

On your exhale, bend your elbows to 90 degrees. Gaze forward, elbows over your wrists, shoulders lowered in line with your elbows. Hug the elbows tight to your ribs and keep your core and legs engaged.

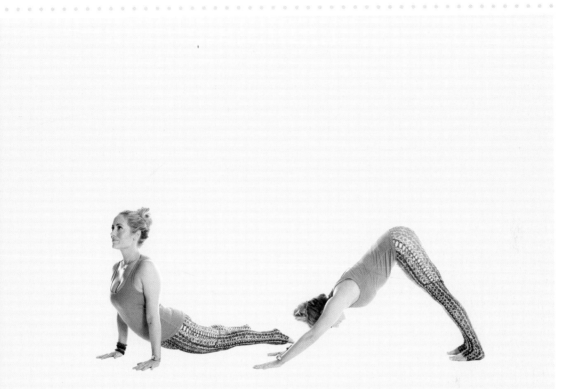

Upward-Facing Dog:
Inhale and flip onto the toenail side of your feet as you drop your hips and straighten your arms. Relax the base of your neck and gently pull your chest through the gateway of your arms. Gaze forward or slightly up.

Downward-Facing Dog:
Exhale and press the ground away as you lift your hips and roll back onto the soles of your feet. Pull your body back into an inverted V shape with your ears in line with your arms, ribs in, legs active and working toward straight.

VINYASA
(PAGES 58–59)

On your exhale, step back into Plank and lower through *Chaturanga*. Inhale into Upward-Facing Dog and exhale into Downward-Facing Dog.

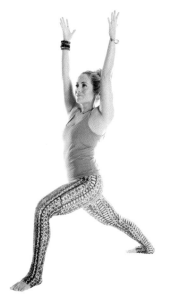

VIRABHADRASANA I (WARRIOR I), SECOND SIDE

INHALE

Step your left foot forward to meet your left thumb and spin your back foot flat so that you have heel-to-heel alignment. Keep your front knee bent as you lift your torso and arms straight up. Square your ribs and hips forward as you continue to root into the outer edge of your back foot. Reach your arms shoulder width apart or draw the palms to touch.

VINYASA (PAGES 58–59)

On your exhale, step back into Plank and lower through *Chaturanga*. Inhale into Upward-Facing Dog and exhale into . . .

ADHO MUKHA SVANASANA
(DOWNWARD-FACING DOG)

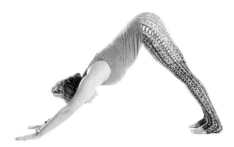

5 BREATHS
Gaze forward at the bottom of your fifth exhale and step or jump to meet your hands.

ARDHA UTTANASANA
(HALF STANDING FORWARD BEND)

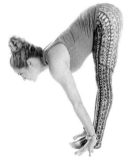

INHALE
Keep your hands down as you extend your torso and gaze forward.

UTTANASANA
(STANDING FORWARD BEND)

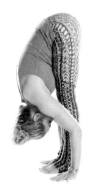

EXHALE
Maintain the length and fold long over your legs.

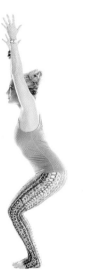

INHALE
Sink your hips and bend your knees as you sweep your arms and torso upright. Keep your front ribs in, hips neutral, and arms reaching up.

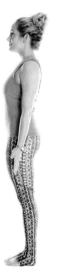

TADASANA
(MOUNTAIN POSE)

EXHALE
Release your arms next to your sides as you straighten your legs.

Welcome to Yoga Routine

This sequence is simple, sweet, and delicious. Nothing overwhelming, but challenging enough to make you stop, think, and even break a sweat. Remember there's no rush and that yoga will always be here for you. You have nothing to prove. Just show up, set your intention, be patient, and have fun!

SUKHASANA (EASY POSE)

1 TO 3 MINUTES

Take a seat on a block. Bend your knees and cross your shinbones at the center, feet landing roughly under your knees. Keep your feet flexed. Sit tall rooting into your tailbone as you lift your sternum and relax your shoulders back. Begin to breathe in and out through your nostrils with the mouth relaxed.

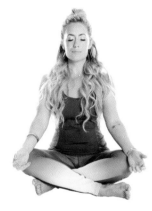

PARIVRTTA SUKHASANA (GENTLE UPRIGHT TWIST)

8 BREATHS PER SIDE

Inhale as you lift tall into your spine. Exhale as you reach your left hand to the outside of your right knee. Place your right fingertips behind your tailbone onto the ground. Focus on lengthening as you inhale and on twisting as you exhale. Keep the hips heavy and revolve from your rib cage. Switch sides and repeat.

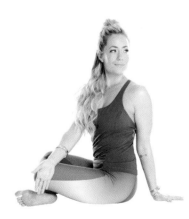

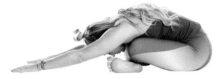

8 BREATHS PER SIDE

Inhale as you lengthen your spine and exhale as you walk your hands forward into a fold. Avoid any rounding in the upper back. Relax your shoulders back. Keep the hips rooted as you extend forward. Take 8 breaths, switch the crossing of your legs, and repeat.

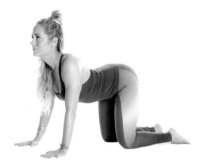

MARJARYASANA-BITILASANA (CAT-COW POSE)

5 ROUNDS

Come onto all fours. Stack your shoulders over your wrists and your hips over your knees. Inhale as you drop your navel, lift your gaze, and roll your shoulders back. Exhale as you round your upper back, push the ground away, and drop your tailbone.

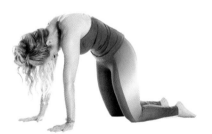

ANAHATASANA
(HEART CHAKRA POSE)

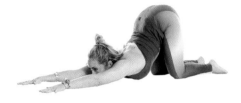

8 BREATHS

Return to all fours. Stack your hips directly above your knees as you walk your arms out in front of you. Melt your heart and belly toward the ground, keeping your gaze forward. Arms stay straight and shoulder width apart. Breathe, and then walk yourself back onto all fours.

ADHO MUKHA SVANASANA
(DOWNWARD-FACING DOG)

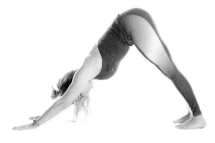

8 BREATHS

Take your hands a few inches forward of your shoulders, curl your toes under, lift your hips and press into your hands to draw your body back into an inverted V shape. Root into your hands to draw energy up the sides of your body as you gently pull your ribs in.

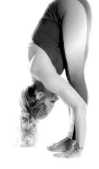

8 BREATHS

Walk your hands back to meet your feet keeping them hip width apart. If there is any strain in your lower back, bend your knees slightly and place your palms on your shins. Otherwise, place your palms on the ground in front of or next to your feet. Lengthen your torso over your thighs, avoiding any rounding in the upper back. Breathe and then walk yourself forward into a pre-push-up position.

PLANK ON KNEES

8 BREATHS

Lower onto your knees and cross your ankles. Keep your arms straight with your shoulders stacking over your wrists, gaze forward. Gently corset your ribs together and lengthen your tailbone. Hold and breathe.

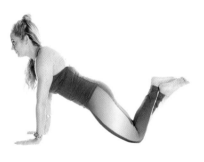

CHATURANGA
(FOUR-LIMBED STAFF POSE) ON KNEES

EXHALE

Keep your gaze forward and bend your elbows to a 90-degree angle. Keep the ribs and sternum extending. Lower to your belly once you complete your breath.

BHUJANGASANA
(COBRA POSE)

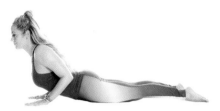

5 BREATHS

Slide your palms back next to your rib cage and release the tops of your feet onto the ground hip width apart. Inhale as you press the ground away and curl your chest and belly button off the mat. Draw your shoulders back and relax through the base of your neck. Gaze forward.

BALASANA
(CHILD'S POSE)

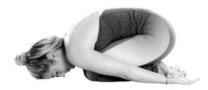

8 BREATHS OR MORE

Drop onto your knees, keeping your legs together. Fold your torso over your thighs and let your forehead rest on the ground with your arms tucked next to your sides like wings. Breathe here for as long as you need.

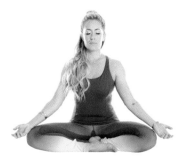

Choose a comfortable way of sitting (cross-legged, propped up on a block, or even in a chair). Rest your hands on your knees, palms facing up for energy or down for focus, or simply cup your palms in your lap. Sit tall with your shoulders relaxed. Close your eyes and slow down your breath. Pick your favorite meditation (pages 243–248) or mantra (page 246) or just enjoy a few moments of quiet.

SAVASANA
(CORPSE POSE)

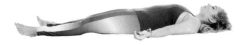

Lie on your back. Gently shake out your arms and legs to release any leftover tension. Snuggle your shoulder blades down the back and let your palms spin up. Rest here for a few minutes or for as long as you desire.

Aim True Routine

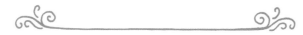

This routine is simple, playful, challenging, and well-rounded. Take a moment to sit quietly or lie on your back and set your intention before you start moving. *Why am I on this mat? What would I like to get out of this practice? How do I want to feel?* Figuring these points out is the key to keeping your aim true even when the going gets tough.

SUN SALUTATION A (PAGES 50–54)

3 ROUNDS

SUN SALUTATION B (PAGES 55–62)

7 ROUNDS

From your last Downward-Facing Dog of round 2, enter this sequence:

VIRABHADRASANA II (WARRIOR II)

8 BREATHS

Step your right foot forward in between your hands. Spin your back heel flat so that the heel of your front foot and the arch of your back foot are aligned. Windmill your arms and torso upright and open. Keep your front knee over your heel. Front ribs stay in as the lower belly lifts. Arms expand actively while the base of the neck relaxes. Gaze forward over your front fingertips. Breathe.

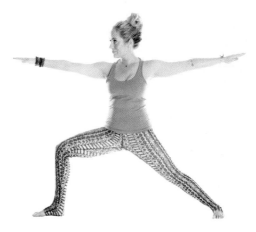

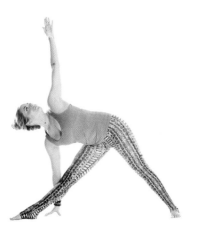

TRIKONASANA
(TRIANGLE)

8 BREATHS

Straighten your front leg as you pull your front hip back. Lengthen through the right side of your waist as you reach forward, landing your hand at the pinky edge of your right foot. Extend your top arm directly overhead. Firm your right hip in as you corset your ribs. Lean your upper body back so that your right side lines up with your right thigh. Breathe.

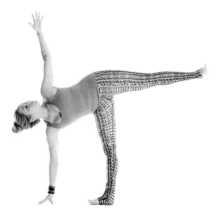

ARDHA CHANDRASANA
(HALF MOON)

8 BREATHS

Place your left hand on your hip and gaze down. Bend your right knee propelling your weight forward onto your right fingertips about a ruler's distance in front of your toes. Draw your left leg up parallel to the ground, keeping it straight and engaged with the toes pointing out. Extend your top arm up to the sky as you hug your rib cage in. Gaze down, sideways, or—for a challenge—up. Breathe.

ARDHA MATSYENDRASANA
(HALF LORD OF FISHES)

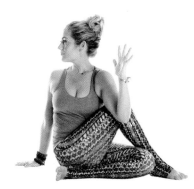

8 BREATHS

Square your hips and place both hands onto the mat. Bend both knees, dropping your left knee behind your right heel to sit down. Inhale and sit tall, reaching your left arm to the sky. Exhale, drop the left arm to the outside of your right thigh, keeping the elbow bent. Place your right hand behind your tailbone on the ground. Inhale as you lengthen, exhale as you push your left arm into your thigh to revolve your chest open. Breathe. Step back into a . . .

VINYASA
(PAGE 58)

Return to Warrior II (page 69) and repeat on the second side. Then move on to . . .

MAKARASANA (DOLPHIN POSE)

3 ROUNDS OF 8 BREATHS EACH

Come onto your knees and place your forearms onto the ground shoulder width apart and parallel. Keep your shoulders over your elbows as you curl your toes under and straighten your legs. Walk your feet in toward your elbows, allowing your hips to lift, but keeping your shoulders stacked above the elbows. Hold for 8 breaths, then release. Rest in between rounds.

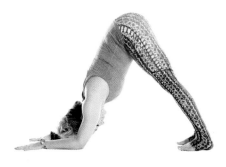

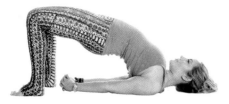

3 ROUNDS OF 8 BREATHS EACH

Lie on your back with both knees bent and the soles of your feet on the ground hip width apart. Lift your hips so you can interlace your fingers underneath your lower back. Rock your shoulders underneath you to broaden the chest. Press into your arms and heels to lift your hips. Keep a slight lift in your chin to keep the neck even and long. Take 8 breaths and rest. Repeat for 3 rounds.

ANANDA BALASANA
(HAPPY BABY)

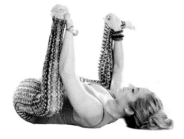

8 BREATHS OR MORE

Lie on your back. Bend both knees and grab hold of your heels from the inside of your legs. Separate your legs wider than hip width apart and let the soles of your feet face up toward the ceiling. Gently draw down on your heels as you relax your shoulders so the thighs descend on either side of your torso. Hold here, breathing, for as long as you like.

AGNISTAMBHASANA
(FIRE LOG OR DOUBLE PIGEON)

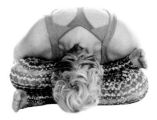

1 TO 5 MINUTES PER SIDE

Roll up to sit. Bend your left knee so that your shinbone faces forward. Cross your right shin onto your left so that the right knee rests above the left foot and your right foot rests above the left knee. Keep both feet flexed. Sit tall or gently lean forward into a fold, eventually resting your forehead on the ground. Switch the crossing of your shins and repeat.

Finish the sequence with a Seated Meditation (page 68) and *Savasana* (page 68).

Empower Routine

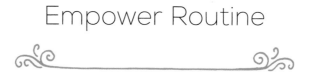

Yoga is a powerful tool to give us confidence regardless of our situation. The poses can serve as a moving prayer or flow of intention. This sequence is made of traditional postures paired with incredible will and drive. Use it anytime you need reminding that your will is stronger than any circumstance or set of opinions.

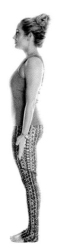

TADASANA
(MOUNTAIN POSE)

5 BREATHS
Take a few deep breaths and set your intention for the practice. Make it clear, and make it yours.

SUN SALUTATION A
(PAGES 50–54)

3 ROUNDS

FIRST ROUND: **Dedicated to Someone You Love**
Think of someone who makes your heart flutter or who immediately puts a smile on your face. Feel the energy of their love

flowing through your entire body. Use this flow as a silent thank-you from your heart to theirs, reminding yourself that love is a two-way street—for every ounce of love and support they've given you, you commit to offering in return.

SECOND ROUND: **Dedicated to Someone Who Has Hurt You**
Think of someone who has hurt you, who constantly triggers your reactive side, or who has left such a scar that you struggle with letting go of the story. Use this salutation to shape your feelings about the person into the form of acceptance and gratitude. Everyone enters our lives for specific reasons. Set your grudges free, thank them for their lessons, and emotionally send them on their way.

THIRD ROUND: **Dedicated to Yourself**
Dedicate this salute to yourself. This is a huge dose of self-love and support. Acknowledge your talents, abilities, and gifts. Embrace exactly who you are in this exact moment in time, noting that you are imperfectly perfect. Love your imperfections as much as the traits you are proud of. Thank your body for having the strength to practice yoga. Smile to yourself as you move thoughtfully through these poses.

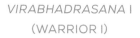

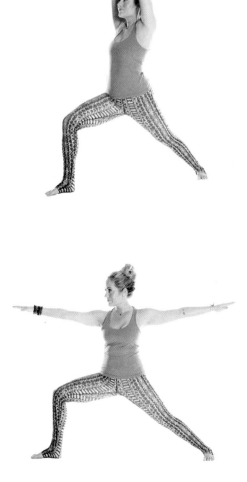

I AM ENOUGH

From Downward-Facing Dog, step your right foot forward next to your right thumb and spin your back foot flat so that the heel of your front foot and the heel of your back foot are aligned. Lift your torso upright, keeping the front knee bent in a 90-degree angle. Work on squaring your hips and torso forward as you extend your arms overhead. Hold for 1 to 5 breaths, telling yourself, "I am enough."

VIRABHADRASANA II
(WARRIOR II)

I AM PERFECTLY IMPERFECT

Toe-heel your right foot over a few inches so that the heel of your front foot and arch of your back foot are aligned as you open your torso. Elevate your arms parallel to the ground and extending away from each other. Keep your front leg at a 90-degree angle. Hold for 1 to 5 breaths as you tell yourself, "I am perfectly imperfect."

VIPARITA VIRABHADRASANA
(REVERSE WARRIOR)

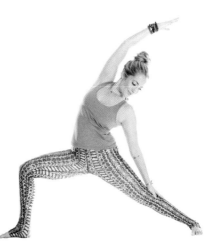

I AM STRONG

Keep the Warrior II stance of your lower body as you rotate your right palm up to the sky. Trickle your left hand down your back leg as you sweep your right hand up and back expanding your side ribs open. Keep the tailbone heavy and the lower belly engaged. Hold for 1 to 5 breaths as you tell yourself, "I am strong."

UTTHITA PARSVAKONASANA
(EXTENDED SIDE ANGLE POSE)

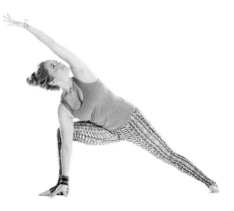

I AM BEAUTIFUL/HANDSOME

Move back through Warrior II, extending your right hand forward and down to the outside of your right foot. Reach your left arm straight up, rotate the palm forward, and extend it overhead. Roll your heart open as you firm your right hip in. Gaze up underneath your arm and breathe for 1 to 5 breaths as you tell yourself, "I am beautiful/handsome."

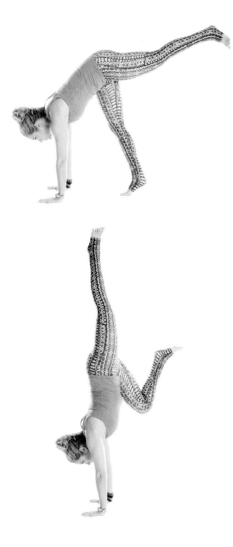

I AM FEARLESS

Come back up to Warrior II. Windmill your hands overhead onto the ground. Pivot to the ball of your back foot and hop your front foot back a few inches. Plant your palms flat shoulder width apart. Firm your arms straight and keep your gaze slightly forward. Lift your left leg up toward the ceiling. Bend your right knee and take a small hop up toward handstand (use a wall if this is new to you), bringing your right knee tight to your chest and working your hips up over your shoulders. Each time, tell yourself, "I am fearless." Take up to 5 hops.

VINYASA
(PAGE 58)

On your exhale, step back into Plank and lower through *Chaturanga*. Inhale into Upward-Facing Dog and exhale into Downward-Facing Dog. Step into Warrior I with the left foot and repeat the sequence on the second side. Then move on to . . .

NAVASANA + ARDHA NAVASANA
(BOAT POSE + HALF BOAT)

5 ROUNDS

Start seated with your knees bent. Hold on to the backs of your thighs as you elevate your feet off the ground balancing on the tripod of your tailbone and two sitting bones. Draw your shinbones parallel to the ground and stay here or keep straightening your legs until your toes are in line with your eyes.

Release your legs and extend your arms straight in line with your shoulders. Hold for 5 breaths.

Lower your body until your legs and shoulder blades hover low over the ground. Extend your arms powerfully straight next to your sides. Gaze at your navel. Hold for 5 breaths. Lift back up into full boat. Repeat, taking five breaths per pose.

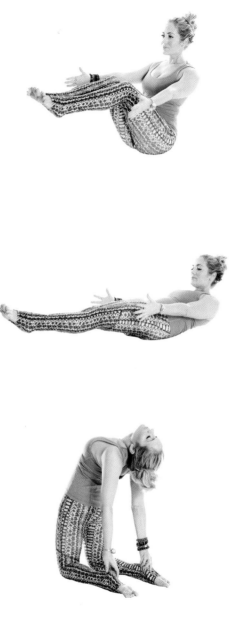

USTRASANA (CAMEL POSE)

3 ROUNDS OF 8 BREATHS EACH

Stand on your knees with even weight throughout your shinbones, keeping them hip width apart, hips stacked over your knees. Drop your tailbone, lift your lower belly, and curl your chest open. Roll your shoulders back and release your head back as you press your heart to the sky. Reach your hands back to grab your heels (or keep them on your hips).

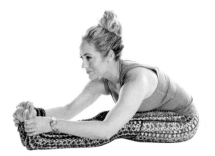

PASCHIMOTTANASANA
(SEATED FORWARD BEND)

Sit with your legs extended straight and together in front of you. Flex your feet. Inhale as you lift your torso tall, exhale as you lengthen your middle long over your legs, grabbing the outer feet or working with a strap over the balls of the feet. Avoid rounding in your spine. Focus on length.

ANANDA BALASANA (HAPPY BABY)

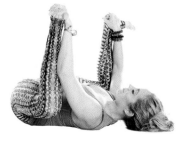

8 BREATHS

Separate your legs wider than hip width apart and let the soles of your feet face up toward the ceiling. Gently draw down on your heels as you relax your shoulders so the thighs descend on either side of your torso. Hold here, breathing, for as long as you like.

RECLINED TWIST

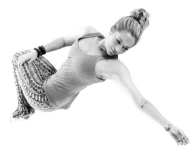

5 BREATHS PER SIDE

Lying on your back, hug your knees into your chest. Open your arms wide and drop both knees over to the right, keeping them stacked. Draw your tailbone forward as you melt your opposite shoulder into the ground. Breathe. Switch sides and repeat.

Finish the sequence with a Seated Meditation (page 68) and *Savasana* (page 68). Place both palms over your heart and thank it for being strong, open, and resilient.

Energize Routine

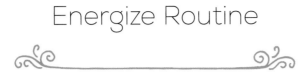

Ever feel so tired and strapped for time that nothing but a bottomless pot of coffee could save you? Cue superhero yoga sequence! This simple (and short) flow of poses is geared to save you time, perk you up, and remind you that you possess all the energy (and pizzazz) of your favorite hero. Go get 'em, tiger!

ANAHATASANA
(HEART CHAKRA POSE)

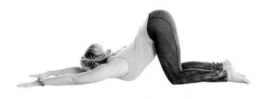

Begin on all fours, with your shoulders stacked over your wrists and your hips over your knees. Keep your hands shoulder width apart and your knees hip width apart. Keep your hips over your knees as you walk your hands forward. Bow your belly and throat down toward the ground until your arms are straight and engaged, fully extended. Keep your hips high, as if you're a puppy wagging its playful tail. Gaze slightly forward as you melt your throat and heart toward the ground.

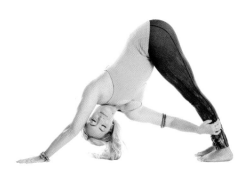

5 BREATHS PER SIDE

Come back onto all fours. Keep your hands slightly forward of your shoulders. Curl your toes under, straighten your legs, and lift your hips up and back into the pose. Firm your upper outer arms in; relax all four sides of your neck. Reach your right hand to the outer edge of your left leg (shin, ankle, or foot, whatever you can reach). If you can't find the leg, shorten your stance. Revolve your rib cage to the left, keeping your left arm straight. Breathe, switch sides, and repeat.

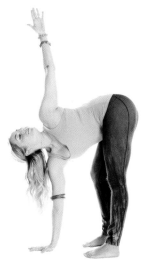

UTTANASANA
(STANDING FORWARD BEND)
WITH TWIST

5 BREATHS PER SIDE

Walk your hands back to meet your feet, keeping them hip width apart. Place your right palm down onto the mat or a block so that your arm is straight, with the shoulder stacking over the wrist. Bend your right knee slightly as you push the ground away and extend your left arm up to the sky. Keep your hips square and relax your neck. Breathe, switch sides, and repeat.

UTKATASANA
(CHAIR POSE)

8 BREATHS

Bend both of your knees, drop your hips, and lift your torso upright. Keep the weight in your heels as you press the shinbones back. You should be able to see your toes when you gaze down. Keep your pelvis neutral, lift your lower belly up, and keep your front ribs in. Extend your arms up shoulder width apart with the palms turned in to relax the base of your neck.

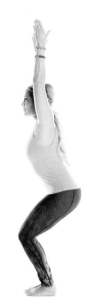

PARIVRTTA UTKATASANA
(CHAIR POSE TWIST)

8 BREATHS PER SIDE

From Chair, draw your palms in to your heart. Exhale, and swing your left elbow onto your right thigh. Place your palms together and press down to revolve your chest open to the right. Keep your hips square. Release the twist, returning into Chair. Repeat the twist on the second side, then place your palms on the ground and step back into . . .

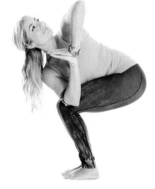

VINYASA
(PAGE 58)

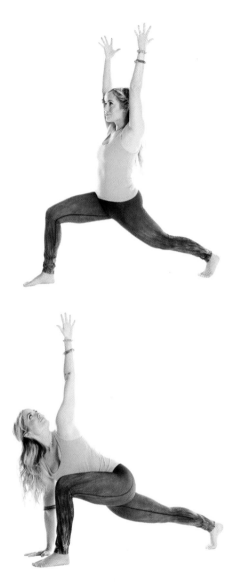

8 BREATHS

Step your right foot forward in between your hands. Stay on the ball of your back foot with your feet hip width apart. Lift your arms and torso upright. Draw your tailbone down as you lift your lower belly up. Bend the back knee as much as you need to in order to achieve this. Stretch your arms overhead shoulder width apart. Breathe.

Drop your left hand down onto the mat, keeping your hips square. Press into your base hand to revolve your chest open to the right, extending your top arm up directly above your left arm. Breathe.

VINYASA
(PAGE 58)

Repeat Crescent + Crescent with hand down twist on the second side.

VINYASA
(PAGE 58)

USTRASANA (CAMEL POSE)

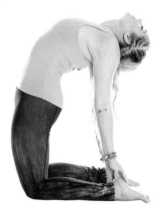

3 ROUNDS OF 8 BREATHS EACH

Hop to your shins. Stand on your knees with even weight throughout your shinbones, keeping them hip width apart. Place your hands on your hips, encouraging your tailbone down and your lower belly up. Shift your hands to your rib cage, inviting it to press forward to create a wheel sensation in your chest. Continue to curl your upper body open as you lift your heart straight up. Release your arms back to clasp your heels. Surrender your neck and head. Breathe, rolling up one vertebra at a time. Repeat.

PASCHIMOTTANASANA
(SEATED FORWARD BEND)

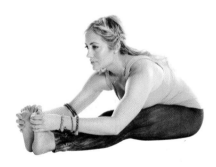

8 BREATHS

Swing your legs out in front of you. Sit tall with your legs straight and together. Flex your feet. Inhale as you lift your chest up. Exhale, keeping the length as you reach forward to grab the outer edges of your feet. Avoid rounding in the upper back. Keep the legs active and the neck soft.

Finish the sequence with a Seated Meditation (page 68) and *Savasana* (page 68). Clear your mind, absorb your practice, and invite energy and renewal into your attitude and body.

Calm Down Routine

This is one of the most delicious nightcaps you can order. Slow, stretchy poses ease your overworked body and mind into a state of calm, happy acceptance of exactly where you are. This routine wrings out your body and aids in clearing out your mind. It may be useful to have a strap or towel for the final poses.

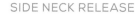

SUKHASANA FOLD

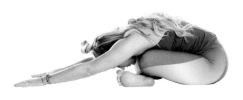

11 BREATHS

Begin in a comfortable cross-legged seated position with your shinbones crossing at the center and your heels flexed under the opposite knees. Sit tall as you inhale and, as you exhale, walk your arms forward, bowing your head to the ground. Keep your spine long. Feel free to place your head onto a block or prop if it doesn't reach the ground. Hold for 11 long breaths. Change the crossing of your legs and repeat.

SIDE NECK RELEASE

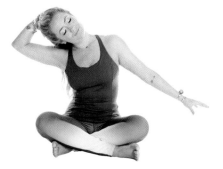

8 BREATHS PER SIDE

Place your right palm on the left side of your head and gently pull down toward the right as you extend your left arm gently out to your side. Keep your left arm engaged and don't worry about landing it on the ground. Change sides and repeat.

15 BREATHS

Open your legs into a wide V shape with your feet flexed. Toes and knees point up to the ceiling. Inhale as you lengthen the spine. Exhale and walk your arms and torso forward as far as you comfortably can without rounding your back. You can place your forehead onto a block.

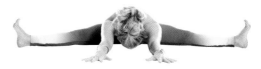

Focus on your inhales and exhales to wash away your day and any distractions.

SIDE STRETCH

11 BREATHS

Stay low and walk your right forearm down to the inside of your right shinbone. Extend your left arm up toward the sky and rotate the palm in. Side-stretch over toward your right foot; if possible, clasp your right foot with your left hand. Revolve your rib cage open and weave your right arm under to clasp the top of your left thigh. Repeat on the second side.

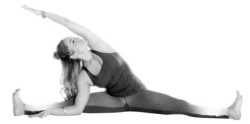

BACK OF THE NECK RELEASE

8 BREATHS

Return your legs to *Sukhasana* and interlace your fingers behind your skull. Hug your elbows in around your face, tuck your chin, round your upper back, and gently pull down on the back of your head.

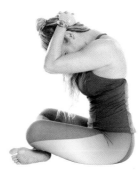

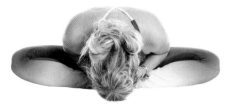

11 BREATHS

Bend both of your knees and bring the soles of your feet together. Draw the heels as far into your groin as you comfortably can. Clasp the outer edges of your feet with your hands and peel the soles of your feet open like a book. Lengthen your spine as you inhale, then exhale, folding forward and reaching your belly toward your feet and your forehead toward the ground. Rest your forehead on a block if you desire.

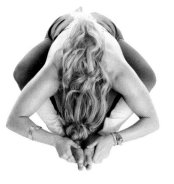

DIAMOND *BADDHA KONASANA*

1 MINUTE

Keep the soles of your feet together, but push them as far away from you as you can without the feet separating. This will create a long diamond shape. Grab the outer edges of your feet and fold forward, reaching your forehead toward your heels. Let your elbows bend wide; relax the base of your neck. Hold here for 1 minute.

RECLINED *PADANGUSTHASANA* (BIG TOE POSE) B

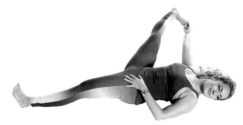

8 BREATHS

Lie on your back and place a strap over the ball of your right foot. Extend your left leg flat on the ground as you extend your right leg straight into the air. Grasp both ends of the strap with your right hand, keeping your shoulders completely relaxed. Rotate your heel in and toes out, then allow your leg to open out to the right. Keep your left hip heavy and shoulders soft. Breathe.

RECLINED *PADANGUSTHASANA* (BIG TOE POSE) C

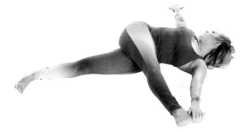

8 BREATHS

Bring your leg back up and switch hands. Begin to drop your right leg over toward the left, keeping it straight and active. Roll your outer thigh forward making more length in your right side. Extend your right arm out to the side and relax it on the ground. Breathe. Return to upright and switch legs.

Finish the sequence with a Seated Meditation (page 68) and/or *Savasana* (page 68).

Self-Love Routine

This sequence is designed to open up your perspective about how your body performs on the mat by reminding it of how perfect and strong it is in every pose. I encourage you to practice this routine solo in your sacred space. Be completely honest with yourself.

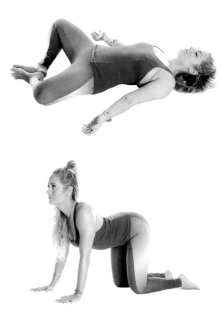

SUPTA BADDHA KONASANA (RECLINING BOUND ANGLE POSE)

Lie on your back with your knees bent and the soles of your feet together. Place your hand on a part of your body that frustrates you or that you dislike. This can be a physical trait ("big thighs," "little arms") or something that symbolizes a character trait (unable to speak up, shortsighted). Hold this part of your body and tell it that you're going to be on the same team. Commit to loving this part of your body and your body as a whole.

MARJARYASANA-BITILASANA (CAT-COW POSE)

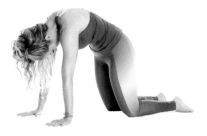

5 ROUNDS

Come onto all fours. Stack your shoulders over your wrists and your hips over your knees. Inhale as you drop your navel, lift your gaze, and roll your shoulders back. Exhale as you round your upper back, push the ground away, and drop your tailbone.

ADHO MUKHA SVANASANA
(DOWNWARD-FACING DOG)

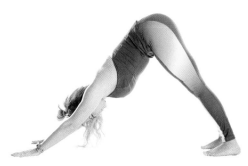

8 BREATHS

Curl your toes under, lift your hips up and back, and straighten your legs as you press firmly into your hands. Spread your fingers evenly and give your head a good shake. *Imagine any unwanted thoughts or negative habits flying out of your mind and splattering on the walls.* Breathe and then walk your hands back to meet your feet and stand.

UTTANASANA
(STANDING FORWARD BEND)

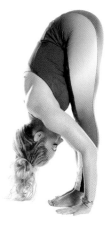

8 BREATHS

Keep your feet hip width apart and grab hold of your forearms as you dangle over your legs. Relax your head completely, but keep your heart extending long toward the ground to avoid rounding in the spine. *Take a few deep breaths here, expelling anger or confusion with your exhales.* Bend both of your knees slightly and drop your arms to the ground. Slowly stack up your spine, one vertebra at a time, to stand, letting your head and chin be the last to roll up.

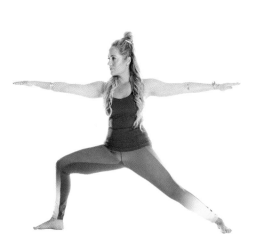

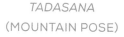

Stand tall at the front of your mat with your feet together. Place both of your palms on top of your heart and bow your gaze down.

Set your intention to aim true in your body and the way you view it. Choose to love it. Let go of the constant battle and sign the treaty to be on the same side. You are strong and vibrant.

VIRABHADRASANA II
(WARRIOR II)

8 BREATHS PER SIDE

Step your right foot forward in between your hands. Spin your back heel flat so that the heel of your front foot and the arch of your back foot are aligned. Windmill your arms and torso up and open. Keep your front knee over your heel. Front ribs stay in as the lower belly lifts. Arms expand actively while the base of the neck relaxes. Gaze forward over your front fingertips. Breathe. *Focus on the incredible power and strength in your thighs. Thank you, legs.* Straighten your front leg, parallel your feet, switch sides, and repeat.

HUMBLE HORSE

8 BREATHS

Keep your feet one leg's distance apart and spin your heels and toes out. Do a few test bends to make sure your knees are pointing in the same direction as your toes. Keep your pelvis neutral and bend your knees, dropping your hips no lower than your knees. Interlace your fingers behind your back and squeeze your arms toward straight. Keep your knees bent as you hinge from your hips and fold your torso forward. Draw your arms up and overhead toward the ground. Hold here.

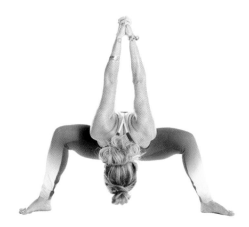

It won't be easy, but your hips and buns are wicked powerful and they are supporting you even when you don't support them with your thoughts. Work that strength!

TWISTER PLANK

Start in Plank pose with your arms straight, shoulders over the heels of your hands, and feet hip width apart. Draw your front ribs in to engage your core and protect your lower back. Inhale and place your right elbow where your right hand is. Follow suit by placing your left elbow where your left hand is, so now you're in Forearm Plank (shoulders directly over the elbows). Reverse this to come back up: right palm where your right elbow is, left palm where your left elbow is. Continue this twister dance from Plank to Forearm Plank and back, keeping your center engaged and your gaze forward for anywhere from 20 seconds to a minute.

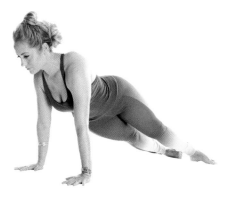

This is a love dance for your belly. The core is the home of experience and love. It's the alarm for truth and honesty and the portal for releasing insecurities (think of butterflies in your stomach). It doesn't need to look a certain way; it just needs to support you and hold you up. Rock that belly.

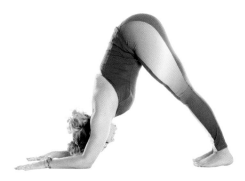

Dear arms, you are impressive. I put you into compromising situations, and you always step up to bat. You help me lift other people up and open me up to love, relationships, and kindness.

MAKARASANA
(DOLPHIN POSE)

3 ROUNDS OF 8 BREATHS EACH

Come onto all fours and place your fore-arms on the ground parallel to each other and shoulder width apart. Curl your toes under and lift your knees off the ground to straighten your legs. Lift your hips and walk your feet in as far as they'll comfort-ably go without shifting your shoulders past your elbows. Breathe.

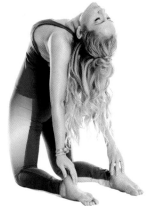

Dedicate this pose to your chest; the home of your heart. Open this space up so you can offer love and accept it in return. Physically manifest the energy you want to project.

USTRASANA
(CAMEL POSE)

3 ROUNDS OF 8 BREATHS EACH

Drop onto your knees with your feet and knees hip width apart. Stand on your knees with even weight throughout your shinbones, keeping them hip width apart, hips stacking over your knees. Drop your tailbone, lift your lower belly, and curl your chest open. Roll your shoulders back and release your head back as you press your heart to the sky. Reach your hands back to grab your heels (or keep them on your hips).

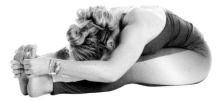

8 BREATHS

Sit down and extend your legs in front of you. Flex your feet and keep the legs together. Inhale as you lengthen your chest, and exhale as you extend forward, reaching for the outer edges of your feet. Avoid any rounding of the upper back, and melt through the base of your neck. Breathe.

THREAD THE NEEDLE

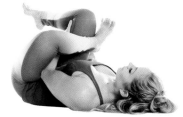

1 TO 2 MINUTES PER SIDE

Lie on your back with your knees bent. Cross your right ankle directly above your left knee and place it on your thigh with your foot flexed. Reach your right arm in between your legs and interlace your fingers behind your hamstring. Gently pull your legs in to stimulate the hip opener. Relax your head on the ground and soften your shoulders. Breathe, switch sides, and repeat.

Come into a comfortable seat and return your hands to the body part you chose at the beginning of class. Give it a supportive squeeze and the commitment that you'll continue to nurture the best possible relationship with it. Sit here in gratitude for 1 to 2 minutes.

Finish the sequence with a Seated Meditation (page 68) and *Savasana* (page 68).

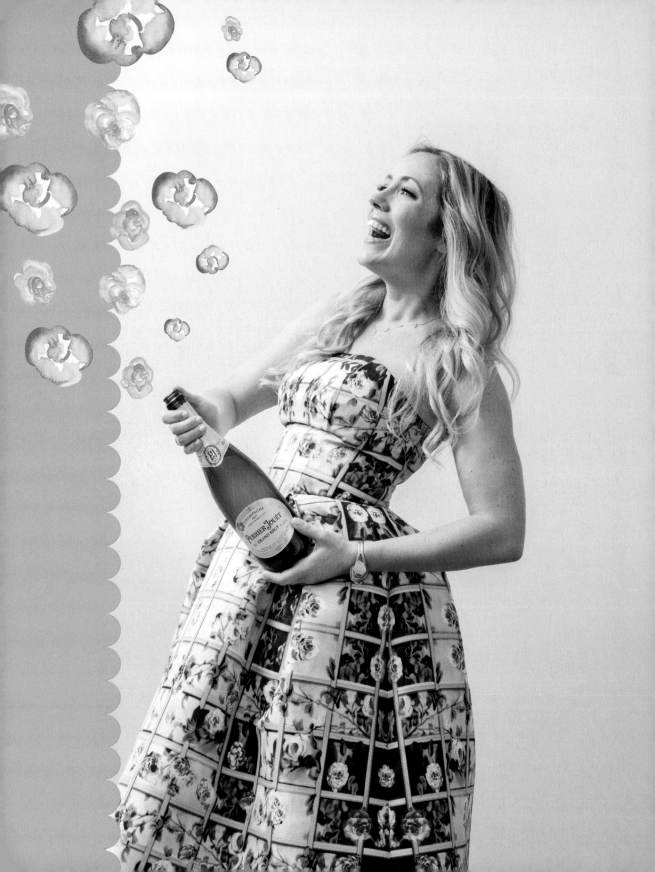

Eat Without Fear

PEOPLE WHO LOVE TO EAT ARE ALWAYS THE BEST PEOPLE.

—Julia Child

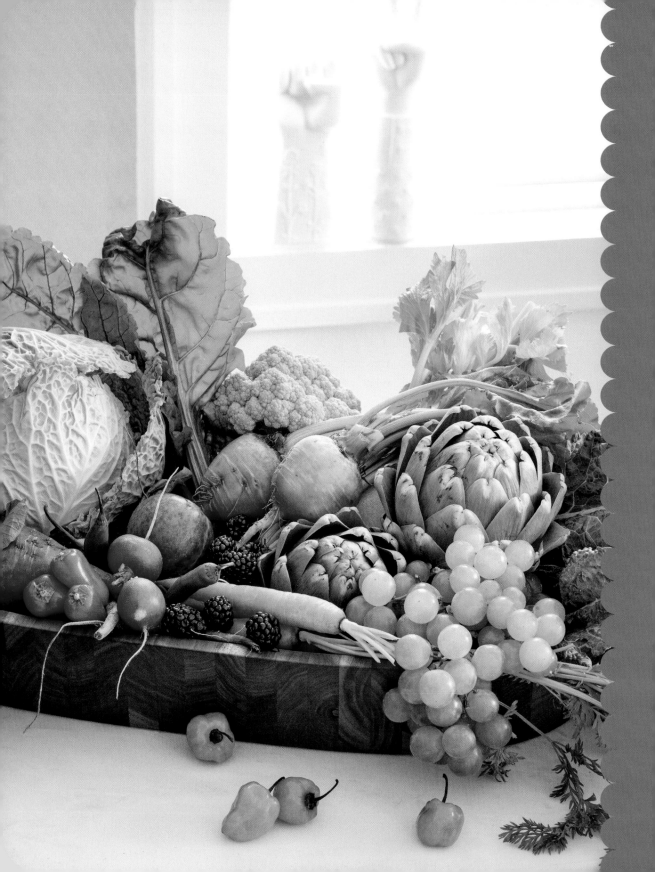

Five

FUEL YOUR BODY

I haven't always been a warrior of health. I grew up in Kansas on a steady diet of Hamburger Helper and thought I was making a healthy choice when I bought the garden vegetable variety of cream cheese. Ah, how things have changed.

It wasn't until I moved to Los Angeles and became immersed in the yoga lifestyle that I had a health epiphany. Suddenly I was surrounded by organic food, amazing healthy restaurants, and fantastic practitioners of health, including Debbie Kim, an acupuncturist, herbalist, and nutritionist. I started seeing her for acupuncture and holistic health appointments that often included discussion about the nutritional choices I was making. Over time, Debbie taught me how to listen to my body, how to care for it as the delicate and powerful vessel that it is, using all of the options I had to keep my mind and body in the best condition possible.

When I started to think about everything Debbie has taught me over the years and how my health has benefited from it, I quickly realized that she was the perfect partner for this chapter on purifying your body. We've worked together as a team to bring you clear and accessible information so that you can move forward confidently while making positive health choices and changes in your life.

The body and its cellular makeup function just like a machine. Think of yourself as a race car. If you don't supply it with good fuel, it isn't going to function well. You need to fuel it properly—with organic, nonprocessed food. Give it the nourishment it desires. Cut out the processed sugars and fillers. Focus on using ample amounts of vegetables, fruits, good fats, and proteins.

Food is the foundation of health, and we can each achieve optimal health by individually assessing our own dietary needs. Every person has a unique genetic makeup, childhood, dietary habits, lifestyle, exercise/exertion levels, and stress patterns, so it only makes sense that we would all have different dietary needs. A qualified health-care professional who works with food sensitivities can help you to figure out your ideal diet. I personally have a mild intolerance to gluten and dairy, and Debbie helped me to realize this and to adjust my diet to take better care of myself. You can also use a simple two-week-elimination challenge: eliminate one common offender ingredient (such as wheat, corn, soy, dairy, or sugar) for two weeks and then reincorporate it into your diet and take note of your body's reaction. You may be pleasantly surprised to find that, after two weeks of being bread-free, your chronic headache has miraculously disappeared.

COMMON FOOD ALLERGIES

Planning a two-week-elimination trial? These common offender ingredients can affect your digestion and well-being.

WHEAT: baked goods, pastas, cereals, thickeners like flour

CORN: tortillas and chips, cereals, thickeners like cornstarch, items that contain corn syrup such as sodas and ketchup

SOY: meat and dairy alternatives, tofu, protein bars and powders

DAIRY: baked goods, cheeses, sauces and dressings, protein powders

SUGAR: desserts and other baked goods, snack foods, sodas and other beverages

Reshape the Way You Look at Food

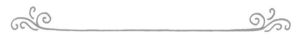

I should make this clear: I love food, and I'm pretty sure it loves me, too.

As I mentioned earlier, I grew up in a land and time where cheese came in the form of a thin orange patty wrapped in plastic, dinner often came out of a box, and I thought Miracle Whip and mayonnaise were the same thing.

Fast-forward to my nutritional enlightenment, and suddenly every piece of food had a story and a purpose—and I realized I was no longer interested in ingesting processed food that's filled with synthetic ingredients. With the education came change, which is a huge part of my passion. I want not only to help people love their food, but to help them understand it, where it comes from and how it serves them. Going from

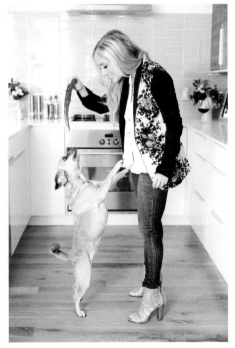

bright orange powdered macaroni and cheese out of the box to white powdered organic mac 'n' cheese out of the box is a small step in the right direction, but what we're working toward is healthy change.

While it's my dream and wish to get everyone to eat better and become educated about where we get our food and how we consume it, I don't want it to consume *us*. You shouldn't feel guilty if you snack on something that came out of a box. It's all about balance.

I must warn you, though—it's easy to get in over your head. Once you board the healthy train, you may find yourself wanting to eat only superfoods. You'll feel guilt if your snack came out of a box or you eat a piece of cheese that isn't organic. This is when I want you to remember the word *balance*.

For example, I have to get photographed. A lot. It's more than is good for the fragile human ego, knowing these images/videos will be seen by a large number of people. This fear trigger used to make me get überstrict with my eating choices anytime I knew I had a photo shoot coming up. This strict diet may have done wonders for my physical body, but it put a major damper on my social life. I couldn't go out to restaurants or meet up with friends for drinks. Travel was almost impossible if I didn't pack all of my own food. It was basically wake up, eat from my diet, work out, go to work, go to sleep, repeat. Not horribly exciting, huh? The moral of that story is I learned what my healthy limits are. I desire optimal health, but I need to balance that with enjoying my life and not feeling guilt about splurging or celebrating from time to time.

My new approach is simple. If I know I need to clean up my act, I make sure to eat protein with every meal. I cut out foods that could cause inflammation, like gluten, dairy, and alcohol. I cut out grains (especially when eating protein) and up my water intake; every day, I focus on having a smoothie with good fats like coconut or flaxseed oil, getting at least eight hours of sleep, meditating, and finding a way to sweat. This is disciplined living, but I'm not depriving myself of a glass of wine if a celebratory push comes to shove. Keep in mind, this is a general way I like to eat, but I don't bash myself if I steer in a different direction. Be healthy, make good choices, but don't feel bad about yourself when you decide you and pizza are majorly overdue for a good date night.

Generally speaking, foods that we want on the best hit list? Major amounts of veg. Debbie recommends that veggies be your best friends. Consume mainly vegetables with a nice complement of fruit, protein, good fats, and carbs.

Try These Healthy Food Swaps

Excited but not really sure where to start? Check out this chart of common foods and their healthier counterparts. How many swaps can you make today?

YOU WON'T EVEN MISS THIS . . .	ONCE YOU TRY THIS!
sodas	sparkling water with lemon, kombucha
breakfast pastries	avocado toast, Quinoa Egg Power Bites (page 134)
white sugar	maple syrup, coconut sugar, raw honey
chips/crackers	gluten-free sesame crackers, kale chips
cow's milk	unsweetened almond milk
cream	coconut milk, cashew cream
white bread	gluten-free bread, sprouted bread
pasta	brown rice pasta, zucchini (vegetable) "noodles"
ice cream	dark chocolate with fresh berries, Cherry Coconut Sorbet with Chocolate and Fresh Herbs (page 221), Maple Cashew Corn-flake Ice Cream (page 223)
bottled salad dressing	all of the easy, homemade dressings in chapter 7, including Vegan Ranch (page 176)
coffee	mate, matcha, green tea
store-bought peanut butter	homemade nut butter

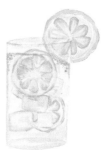

THE CLEANSE EVERYONE
CAN AND SHOULD DO

Drinking water may seem like a no-brainer, but most people live in a constant state of dehydration. Water is pivotal to your physical health, your complexion, and even your body weight. It can actually help you lose weight, as it's an appetite suppressant if you drink it before eating, it boosts your metabolism, and it helps flush toxins from your body.

Commit to the ultimate cleanse: drink eight glasses of water a day. Start every day with one to two large glasses of room-temperature water; you can add the juice of half a lemon if it helps you get it down. This ritual will wake up your digestive system faster than coffee! It is the perfect way to stay regular.

Don't crave water? Spice up your water life by buying a sparkling water maker. Add a dash of lemon or lime juice, and it's incredibly refreshing. You'll find yourself drinking more.

The 5-Day Purification Process

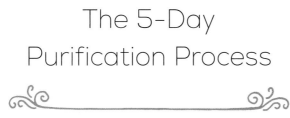

One of the most valuable things Debbie has taught me is that a purification process (what others may refer to as a cleanse or detox) can be a glorious recharge button that wipes the slate clean of any unwanted graffiti that cover your true masterpiece. When someone does a more traditional cleanse, they may live off juice for ten days, only to go bulldozing back into a burrito because they've felt so deprived. A purification process doesn't deprive you—it simply gives your regular eating choices a much-needed makeover.

This five-day purification features five meals a day that you can drink *and* chew—and it even includes snacks! I recommend using all organic ingredients and fresh herbs when and if possible. For recommended protein powders, check out "A Few of My Favorite Things" on page 311.

Debbie Kim's #1 rule to a successful purification process is this: Take it *slow*. Be sure to do that. The recipes in the process are quick and easy, but they do require daily cooking. Switching up your routine may not be convenient or easy, but it's one of the best ways to wipe the system and reboot in order to perform to your ultimate ability. If that doesn't fit with your schedule right now, focus on adding more servings of vegetables to your daily diet. Think of the purification process as a way to truly connect with what you're putting into your body and how it makes you feel. Ideally, you'll feel so much better that you will start craving the clean food from the purification process!

DAY 1

BREAKFAST

Fresh Herb Omelet

MAKES 1 SERVING

Shave 1 zucchini into wide ribbons with a peeler and blanch it in boiling water for 30 seconds. Remove the ribbons from the water and pat dry. Heat 1 tablespoon extra-virgin olive oil in a frying pan over medium heat. Arrange the zucchini strips on the pan to cover the entire bottom. Crack 2 eggs into a bowl and whisk. Pour them over the zucchini strips and sprinkle on ½ teaspoon sea salt, ¼ teaspoon black pepper, and 1 tablespoon chopped tarragon or mint. Fry the omelet for 3 to 4 minutes. Flip half of the zucchini base over the other side to create an omelet. Fry until golden, or another 2 minutes per side.

SNACK

Raspberry Smoothie

MAKES 1 SMOOTHIE

Combine ¼ cup protein powder, 1 cup frozen raspberries, 1 cup coconut milk, 2 teaspoons raw honey, and 1 teaspoon coconut oil in a blender. Blend until smooth.

Wild Arugula and Peach Salad

MAKES 1 SERVING

Wash and slice ½ peach. Combine it with 1 cup wild arugula and ¼ avocado, diced. For the dressing, mix 1 tablespoon extra-virgin olive oil, 1 tablespoon apple cider vinegar, 1 minced shallot, 2 teaspoons Dijon mustard, and 1 pinch of sea salt.

Roasted Cauliflower Soup

MAKES 2 TO 4 SERVINGS

Preheat the oven to 450°F. Remove the leaves from 1 head cauliflower and break up the head into florets. Toss them with 2 tablespoons extra-virgin olive oil, 2 teaspoons red pepper flakes, and 2 teaspoons sea salt. Roast for 30 minutes, mixing occasionally. Sauté 1 chopped leek, 2 chopped carrots, 2 chopped celery stalks, and 3 minced shallots in 1½ tablespoons ghee or butter for 10 minutes. Add 4 cups chicken or vegetable broth and simmer for another 10 minutes. Taking care with the hot vegetable mixture, use a blender to puree it, along with three-quarters of the roasted cauliflower, until smooth. Top the soup with the remaining cauliflower florets.

SNACK

Classic Green Smoothie

MAKES 1 SMOOTHIE

Blend 1 cup kale, 1 cup romaine, ½ apple, 1-inch piece peeled fresh ginger, the juice of ½ lemon, a handful of basil, 1 tablespoon coconut/omega/flaxseed oil, and 1 cup raw or unsweetened coconut water until smooth.

Herbed Quinoa

MAKES 2 SERVINGS

Soak 1 cup white quinoa in water for 1 hour or overnight and drain (see Sidebar page 153). In a large saucepan, combine the quinoa with 2 cups vegetable or chicken broth, 1 tablespoon ghee or butter, and 2 teaspoons sea salt. Bring to a boil, stir well, and reduce heat to maintain a low simmer for 10 to 15 minutes, or until the grains are fluffy. Brown ½ pound ground light meat turkey (if desired), and drain. For the dressing, combine 2 tablespoons extra-virgin olive oil, the juice of 1 lemon, 1 tablespoon chopped basil, 1 tablespoon chopped flat-leaf parsley, 1 tablespoon chopped thyme, and 2 teaspoons sea salt. Place the quinoa and turkey into a serving bowl, pour the dressing over them, and mix well.

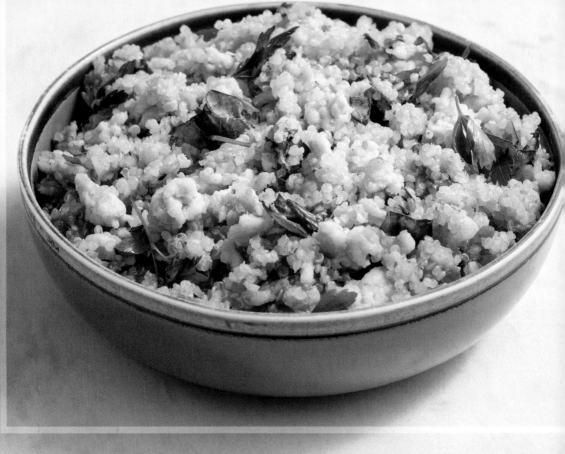

Steamed Broccoli with Lemon-Nutritional Yeast Dip

MAKES 2 SERVINGS

In a large pot, bring about 3 inches of water to a boil and steam 1 head of broccoli in a steamer for 5 to 10 minutes, or until bright green. For the dip, mix 2 tablespoons extra-virgin olive oil, the juice of 2 lemons, 5 tablespoons nutritional yeast, and 2 teaspoons sea salt.

DAY 2

BREAKFAST

Egg Scramble

MAKES 1 SERVING

Beat 2 eggs and combine them with ½ cup sliced mushrooms, ½ cup diced tomato, and 2 cups spinach. Melt 1 tablespoon ghee or butter in a frying pan over medium-high heat. Add the egg mixture and stir constantly until the eggs are fully cooked, about 3 minutes. Top with ¼ avocado, diced. Salt to taste.

SNACK

Citrus Smoothie

MAKES 1 SMOOTHIE

Combine ¼ cup protein powder, 3 cups spinach leaves, 1 peeled orange, ½ cup water, 10 green grapes, 1 tablespoon coconut oil, and 1 thin slice of lime plus the juice from the remainder of the lime in a blender. Add a handful of ice cubes and blend until smooth.

Steamed Artichoke with Lemon Butter

MAKES 1 SERVING

Steam 1 artichoke for 1 hour and 15 minutes. Melt 2 tablespoons ghee or butter with the juice of 1 lemon. Add a pinch of sea salt and use this lemon butter as a dip for the artichoke leaves and heart.

Tomato Fennel Soup

MAKES 2 TO 4 SERVINGS

Heat 2 tablespoons extra-virgin olive oil in a large saucepan over medium heat and sauté 2 sliced fennel bulbs, 3 minced garlic cloves, and 1 teaspoon red pepper flakes for 5 to 7 minutes, or until the fennel is soft. Add 2 cups halved cherry tomatoes and 2 teaspoons sea salt. Sauté for another 10 minutes, or until the tomatoes are wilted. Cover with 4 cups vegetable or chicken broth and simmer for 15 minutes. Combine in a high-speed blender with 2 tablespoons light coconut cream (scooped from the solid part of a can of coconut milk). Top with a handful of slivered basil.

SNACK

Classic Green Smoothie

See page 107.

DINNER

Roasted Fish

MAKES 1 SERVING

Preheat the oven to 375°F. Place 1 fillet of salmon or white fish (sole or tilapia, for example) in an oversized piece of parchment paper. Cover it with 1 tablespoon extra-virgin olive oil, 2 teaspoons minced fresh thyme, 2 teaspoons minced flat-leaf parsley, 1 minced garlic clove, ½ cup diced canned San Marzano tomatoes, and 1 teaspoon sea salt. Fold the paper over the fillet to make a pocket, overlap the paper, crimp the edges to seal, and bake for 20 minutes.

ROASTED FISH
(PAGE 110)

Sautéed Garlic Kale

MAKES 2 SERVINGS

Wash 1 bunch kale, then remove and discard the ribs; mince 3 garlic cloves. In a large saucepan over medium heat, heat 2 tablespoons coconut oil and sauté the garlic for 2 minutes. Add the kale and sauté for another 3 to 4 minutes, or until it is wilted but still maintains its color. Sprinkle with sea salt to taste.

DAY 3

. . . .

BREAKFAST

Asian Bowl

MAKES 1 SERVING

Place ½ cup cooked brown rice in a bowl and drizzle it with 1 tablespoon tamari. Steam 2 bunches of bok choy for 5 minutes and place it on top of the rice. Bring 1 cup water to a boil and add 1 tablespoon white miso paste. Stir well and boil for 5 minutes. Fry 1 egg in 1 teaspoon coconut oil for 3 minutes over medium heat, or until the white is cooked through. Pour the miso over the rice, then top it with the egg and 1 tablespoon chopped scallions (white and green parts).

SNACK

Fresh Smoothie

MAKES 1 SMOOTHIE

Combine ¼ cup protein powder, 2 cups spinach leaves, ½ cucumber, the juice of 1 lemon, a 1-inch piece peeled fresh ginger, ½ apple, ¼ cup fresh pineapple chunks, 1 tablespoon coconut oil, 1 cup water, and a handful of mint in a blender and blend until smooth.

LUNCH

Quinoa with Butternut Squash

MAKES 2 SERVINGS

Soak 1 cup red quinoa in water for 5 minutes and drain (see Sidebar page 153). Combine the quinoa with 2 cups chicken or vegetable broth, 1 tablespoon ghee or butter, and 2 teaspoons sea salt in a large pot. Bring it to a boil. Stir well, then reduce the heat to maintain a low simmer. Add ½ cup cubed butternut squash and cook, covered, for 10 to 15 minutes, or until fluffy. Serve it over a bed of raw spinach with a light sprinkling of paprika and sea salt and a drizzle of extra-virgin olive oil. Add 1 cup skinless rotisserie chicken, if desired.

Mushroom Soup

MAKES 2 TO 4 SERVINGS

Heat 2 tablespoons ghee or butter in a frying pan over medium heat. Add 5 chopped shallots, 2 minced garlic cloves, and 2 teaspoons sea salt and sauté for 5 minutes. Add 2 cups mixed chopped mushrooms and 1 tablespoon chopped fresh sage. Sauté for another 5 minutes. Add 4 cups vegetable or chicken broth and simmer for 15 minutes. Using a blender, carefully puree the soup until smooth.

SNACK

Classic Green Smoothie

See page 107.

Maple-Roasted Brussels Sprouts Bowl

MAKES 2 TO 4 SERVINGS

Bring 1 cup brown rice and 2 cups chicken or vegetable broth to a boil with 1 tablespoon ghee or butter and 2 teaspoons sea salt. Stir, reduce the heat to low, cover the pot, and cook for 20 minutes, or until the rice is fully cooked and fluffy. Preheat the oven to 425°F. Toss 2 cups halved Brussels sprouts with 2 tablespoons coconut oil, 2 tablespoons maple syrup, 2 tablespoons Dijon mustard, and 3 diced shallots. Place on a baking sheet and roast for 30 minutes, or until slightly brown. Toss with the rice.

DAY 4

BREAKFAST

Fried Egg with Sweet Potato Hash

MAKES 1 SERVING

Melt 1 tablespoon coconut oil in a frying pan over medium-high heat and add 1 cup diced sweet potatoes. Sprinkle with 1 teaspoon seasoned salt and 1 teaspoon paprika. Cook for 10 to 15 minutes, or until the potatoes are soft and slightly browned. Shortly before the potatoes are done, melt 1 more teaspoon coconut oil in another frying pan over medium-high heat. Crack 1 egg into the pan and let it fry for 3 minutes or until the white is cooked through and the yolk is the desired consistency. Serve the egg on top of the hash.

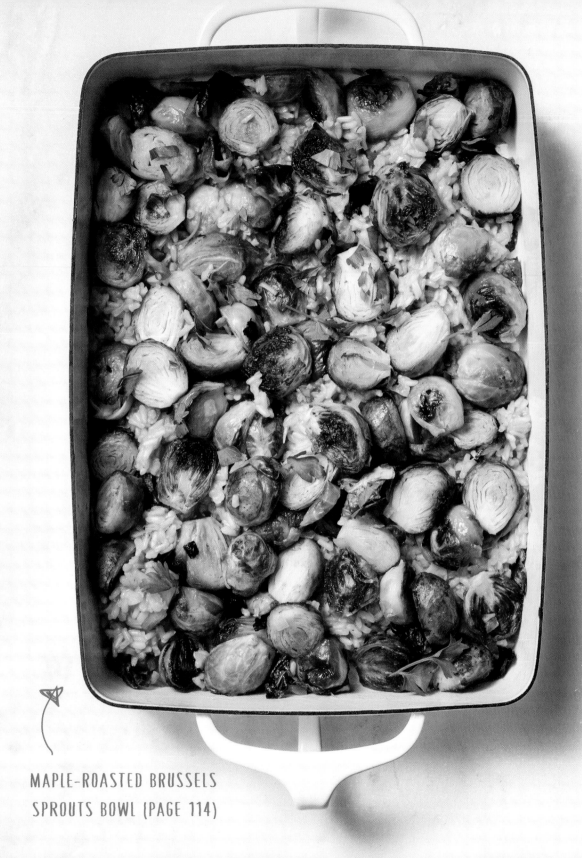

MAPLE-ROASTED BRUSSELS
SPROUTS BOWL (PAGE 114)

Orange Sky Juice

MAKES 1 SERVING

Blend 2 carrots, strain the juice, and return it to the blender. Add ¼ cup protein powder, 1 peeled orange, a 1-inch piece peeled and minced fresh ginger, 1 cup coconut water, and 1 tablespoon coconut oil. Blend until smooth.

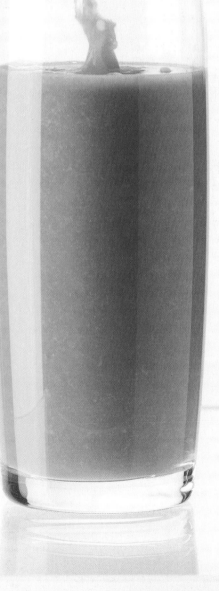

Kale Salad

MAKES 2 SERVINGS

Wash 1 bunch kale; remove and discard the ribs. Tear the kale leaves into pieces and place them in a large bowl; massage them with 1 tablespoon extra-virgin olive oil and 1 teaspoon sea salt and let the salad sit for 10 minutes. Sprinkle it with 2 tablespoons dried cranberries, 1 tablespoon apple cider vinegar, and a pinch of black pepper. Mix well.

Asparagus Soup

MAKES 2 TO 4 SERVINGS

Remove and discard the woody parts, then chop 1 bunch asparagus. In a frying pan over medium-high heat, melt 2 tablespoons ghee or butter and sauté 1 diced sweet onion, 2 garlic cloves, and 2 teaspoons sea salt for 8 to 10 minutes, or until the onion is soft. Add the chopped asparagus and cook for another 5 minutes. Cover with 4 cups chicken or vegetable broth and sauté for 15 minutes. Transfer the soup to a blender, carefully puree it until smooth, and season to taste.

SNACK

Classic Green Smoothie
See page 107.

Salmon Burgers

MAKES 2 SERVINGS

Blitz ½ pound cold wild salmon in a food processor until the fish is well ground. Transfer it to a large bowl. Add ¼ red onion, chopped, ¼ cup roughly chopped flat-leaf parsley, 2 tablespoons roughly chopped capers, zest of ½ lemon, ½ teaspoon lemon juice, ½ tablespoon extra-virgin olive oil, and 1 teaspoon sea salt. Mix it well with your hands and form it into 2 patties. Heat a grill pan over medium-high heat and spray it with coconut oil. Grill the patties for 3 to 4 minutes on each side. Serve the patties sandwiched between red-leaf lettuce leaves. Add a drizzle of Lemon–Nutritional Yeast Dip (page 109).

DAY 5

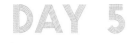

BREAKFAST

Baked Avocado Egg

MAKES 1 SERVING

Preheat the oven to 425°F. Halve 1 avocado and remove the pit and a bit of meat from the center of each half. Lightly salt the avocado and place each half into a small ramekin. Crack 2 small eggs, placing one into each avocado half. Bake for 20 to 25 minutes, or until the egg whites are cooked. Season with sea salt and black pepper to taste and add fresh herbs (such as chives, parsley, cilantro).

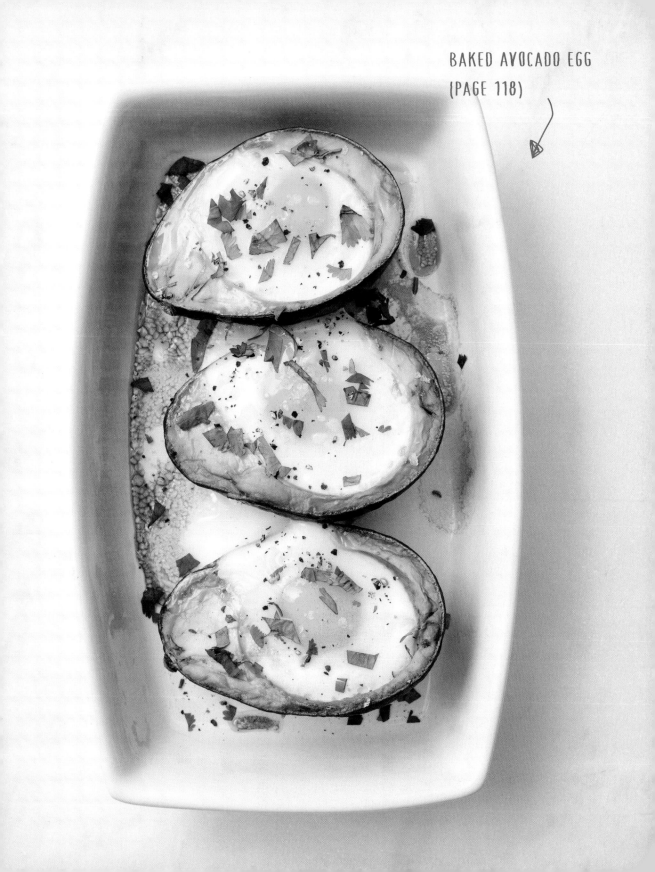

BAKED AVOCADO EGG
(PAGE 118)

Apple Pie Smoothie

MAKES 1 SERVING

Combine ¼ cup protein powder, 1 apple, 1 tablespoon apple cider vinegar, 1 cup water, 2 teaspoons cinnamon, 1 tablespoon raw honey, 1 tablespoon coconut oil, and the juice of 1 lemon in a blender. Blend until smooth.

LUNCH

Crunchy Root Salad

MAKES 1 SERVING

Finely slice or shave 3 radishes, ¼ yellow beet, ¼ red beet, ½ fennel bulb, 1 apple, and 1 carrot. Mix well and place over a bed of radicchio and arugula. For the dressing, combine 2 tablespoons extra-virgin olive oil, 2 tablespoons apple cider vinegar, 1 tablespoon lime juice, 1 minced garlic clove, and 2 teaspoons chopped fresh tarragon. Drizzle the dressing over the salad.

Carrot Soup

MAKES 2 TO 4 SERVINGS

In a frying pan over medium-high heat, melt 2 tablespoons ghee or butter. Add 2 minced garlic cloves, 1 diced sweet onion, 2 chopped celery stalks, 5 chopped carrots, and 1 teaspoon red pepper flakes and sauté for 10 minutes. Drizzle 1 tablespoon maple syrup over the vegetables and sauté for another 3 minutes. Add 4 cups vegetable broth and simmer for 15 minutes. Stir in ¼ cup canned light coconut milk. Transfer the soup to a blender and carefully puree it until smooth.

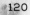

Classic Green Smoothie

See page 107.

Stuffed Bell Peppers

MAKES 4 SERVINGS

Preheat the oven to 375°F. Bring 1 cup jasmine rice to a boil in 2 cups chicken broth, 2 teaspoons sea salt, and 1 tablespoon ghee or butter. Stir well, reduce the heat to low, and cover the pot for 20 minutes, or until the rice is fluffy. In a frying pan over high heat, brown ½ pound ground buffalo or turkey with 1 teaspoon seasoned salt. Dice 1 mango and stir it into the meat. Chop the tops off 4 red bell peppers, remove the seeds and membranes, and fill the peppers with the rice and meat mixture. Place them in a baking pan and roast for 20 minutes.

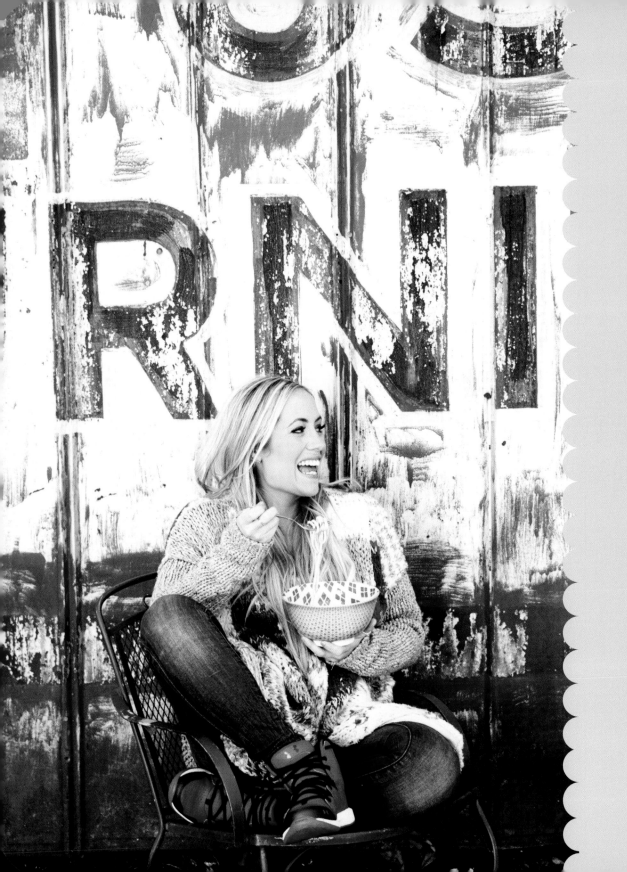

Six

MEALS ARE MEANT
to Be ENJOYED

My absolute favorite food in the world is pasta. White-flour-based, gluten-filled pasta. That's right, a food with virtually no health benefits and a nightmare for anyone with a wheat allergy or sensitivity. I continue to admit it loud and proud—pasta is my love and my Achilles' heel.

Now, consider this: I'm sitting at a restaurant, famished, and I flip the menu open to be faced with two dramatically different choices. On one page they're featuring the daily special: *delicious pasta!* A mountain of noodles swimming in one of my favorite sauces accompanied by nothing green or of any sort of nutritional value. The flip page offers me something quite different—steamed kale, lentils, no sauce. Straight-up medicinal food that will fuel me, nourish me, and make me feel complete, yet . . .

The pasta! The pasta will make my belly sing for joy, beg for more, ask to be whisked away to Italy where we can live happily ever after. Meanwhile the kale and lentils are wooing me with their health benefits, and I know I'll digest them well. The pasta might make me feel fat and bloated, but the kale still can't hold a candle to it.

Do I want to stay healthy or go all out? Do I behave and eat the kale, or is it okay to splurge and have the pasta? This debate continues in my mind until the waiter arrives at the table, at which point I gaze up with confused doe eyes. To be healthy or not to be healthy—is that the question? Here's my answer: order the freakin' pasta.

Our lives are short and sweet, and how tragic would it be if you ordered the kale only to get hit by a car on your way home with your last thought being, *Why didn't I order the paaaaasssstaaaa?!*

I want you to be a warrior of health, but I want you to balance that out with being a warrior of balance and love. Eating a bowl of pasta (or whatever your favorite food is) bears no shame. Our taste buds exist to be awoken and tantalized! Food provides a symphony of flavors to experience, remember, and relish. When you order or prepare your favorite food, you're treating your belly, heart, and soul. It's a simple treat to reward your body for showing up every day and allowing you to function properly. This is how I want you to view food—as the beautiful gift that it is. Clearly, food is here to nourish us and keep us alive. I also believe we can use it as medicine—to heal our bodies naturally and fully. I also view food as a platform to create friendships, bonds, and alliances, and as an unspoken way to share joy, passion, and love.

How You View Your Food

A huge number of food neuroses come from the emotions we project onto food. I joke about my Dr. Jekyll and Mr. Hyde conversation over pasta versus kale, but this isn't as uncommon as you might think. We're taught that certain foods will make us fat, while others will make us skinny. Once you have this association with foods (think of words like *fat, oil, butter*), you steer far away from them so as to not experience the guilt of crossing over onto the dark side. It always feels good to plow into a pint of ice cream, but afterward we often sit remorsefully rubbing our soft (but happy) bellies.

My question is this: what if we could eat food without regret? What if we could drop the labels associated with certain types of food and just view them as experiences? When you associate a specific food with negativity and fear, it takes on that energy. For example, if you want to eat a chocolate chip cookie, but your guilty conscience is weighing you down, it will be a horrible experience. You'll eat the cookie, crying on the inside, knowing each bite will add an unwanted bulge some-where. At this point, what's the purpose in even eating the cookie? There's no enjoyment, just judgment and pain, when all you wanted was the simple pleasure of eating a cookie.

This negativity infuses the food, and this attitude (whether we're convinced we can't eat something or that a bite of something will send us off the deep end) makes us physically and emotionally sick. We have the power to change this by altering the way we look at food. You can sit down with that cookie and realize with a knowing smile that this cookie might be one of the highlights of your day. All those small little chips of chocolaty goodness are going to give your belly a hug. They might even throw a dance party in your stomach once they get there. Point being, it's going to rock. Next thing you know, you've eaten a "bad" food with a loving attitude, and guess what? You feel fine. Actually, you feel great. Guilt-free, satisfied, and satiated.

My caveat to this would be don't live off a steady diet of cookies. It's still crucial to eat smart and to have balance in everything that you do. There's the famous joke, "I do everything in moderation, except moderation." While this always puts a smile on my face, moderation is key. You're out to dinner—order some pasta. Special occasion—have the cake. Celebrating—drink up! Day-to-day basis? Be smart. Eat organic nonprocessed foods. Choose colorful foods full of nutrients to heal and fuel your body. Want a glass of wine (or two) with your beautiful, nutritious meal? Cheers to your health and sweet, sweet balance.

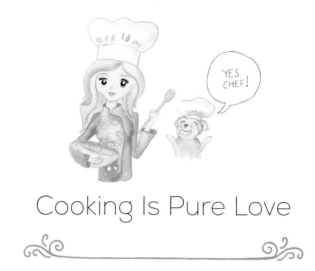

Cooking Is Pure Love

I want you to love your food without fear. I've filled this book up with tons of healthy recipes inspired by all of my teachers, travels, and experiences to make your life easier and more delicious. Whether you make dinner at home on the regular or use your oven for sweater storage (bless your water-boiling heart), it's time to listen up and seduce your inner chef.

My magical cooking abilities weren't inherited—they were learned. I've grown from an artificial-cheese-nibbling girl to a classic-meat-sauce-making teenager (with the help of a boyfriend's parents who taught me the basics) to an enchiladas-for-the-masses-wielding collegian to a health-savvy yogi and, finally, to a balanced home chef influenced and mentored by the pros. I taught chef Giada De Laurentiis private yoga regularly for years; we would stretch, strengthen, and talk about everything and anything food. Giada answered all my questions, from what I should cook on a first date to how to make the perfect birthday cake and why you should never, ever date a chef (even if he's gorgeous). Her encouragement and tutelage pushed my cooking from a mere hobby to a full-on love affair.

This journey has not only expanded the ingredients in my pantry, it's opened my mind and heart. Cooking is a direct gateway to the heart, but it's also the highway to health.

Let's make a short intention list of how we're going to aim true in the kitchen:

✔ Consume fresh produce daily.

✔ Buy organic food whenever possible.

✔ When consuming meat, buy grass-fed, free range, and humane meat. Your best bet is the local farmers' markets. Eat something green every day (something alive, that is—not M&M's).

✔ Drink ample amounts of water (aim for at least eight glasses per day).

✔ Commit to having at least three meals per week where you sit down, free of distractions, and enjoy your meal with yourself or loved ones.

✔ Experiment with one new recipe per week.

5 Ways to Serve Up
Love on a Plate in a Pinch

The actual act of cooking is about as cathartic as it gets, and the act of feeding people? It's pure love. You might love to cook but find you never have the time. Here are five easy solutions to a busy schedule when you still want good, delicious food.

Easy Creamy Quinoa

MAKES 2 TO 4 SERVINGS

In a saucepan, combine 1 cup quinoa (see Sidebar page 153) with 2 cups water or broth, a dash of extra-virgin olive oil, and a pinch of sea salt. Bring to a boil, then reduce the heat and cook for 10 to 15 minutes, or until fluffy. Set the pan aside, covered. Blend 1 (15-ounce) can garbanzo beans, 1 (13.5-ounce) can light coconut milk, 2 chopped garlic cloves, ¼ cup extra-virgin olive oil, 2 teaspoons sea salt, and 1 teaspoon cumin until smooth. Pour this sauce over the quinoa and garnish with cilantro and red pepper flakes.

Cynthia's Baked Fish

MAKES 4 SERVINGS

Preheat the oven to 375°F. Combine ½ cup soy-free vegan mayo, 2 tablespoons Dijon mustard, the juice of 1 lemon, 1 tablespoon Old Bay seasoning, and 2 teaspoons sea salt. Dip 4 (4-ounce) fillets white fish (such as tilapia, cod, or turbot) into the dressing and then coat them with gluten-free panko bread crumbs. Place them on a baking sheet lined with tin foil and spray them with coconut oil. Bake them for 6 to 8 minutes, or until they are flaky and golden brown.

Aim True

Cilantro Fried Eggs

MAKES 1 TO 2 SERVINGS

Warm 2 tablespoons coconut oil in a frying pan. Crack 2 eggs into the pan. Season with 2 teaspoons turmeric and 1 teaspoon sea salt. Sprinkle with fresh cilantro. Fry until the whites solidify and then flip the eggs over for 20 seconds. Serve alone or as a sandwich on toasted buttered bread.

Almond Sauce Curry

MAKES 4 SERVINGS

Cook 12 ounces brown rice pasta to al dente, following the package directions, and drain. Meanwhile, combine the following in a blender: 1 (13.5-ounce) can light coconut milk, 2 tablespoons almond butter, 1 tablespoon curry powder, 1 tablespoon chili powder, 1 teaspoon paprika, 3 garlic cloves, 2 tablespoons tomato paste, 1 teaspoon turmeric, a 1-inch piece peeled fresh ginger, ½ teaspoon cinnamon, 3 tablespoons hot sauce, a pinch of cayenne, and 2 teaspoons sea salt. Puree until smooth and pour over the drained noodles. Add 3 cups raw or sautéed spinach and serve.

Lemon Chicken Wraps

MAKES 1 SERVING

Remove the meat from a store-bought rotisserie chicken. Make Lemon Vegan Mayo (page 210). Heat 1 tablespoon coconut oil in a frying pan over medium-low heat and add a large brown rice or gluten-free tortilla. Warm each side of the tortilla for about 45 seconds, or until slightly golden. Spread the lemon mayo onto the tortilla, add a handful of wild arugula, 1 slice tomato, and ½ cup of the chicken. Roll up and enjoy!

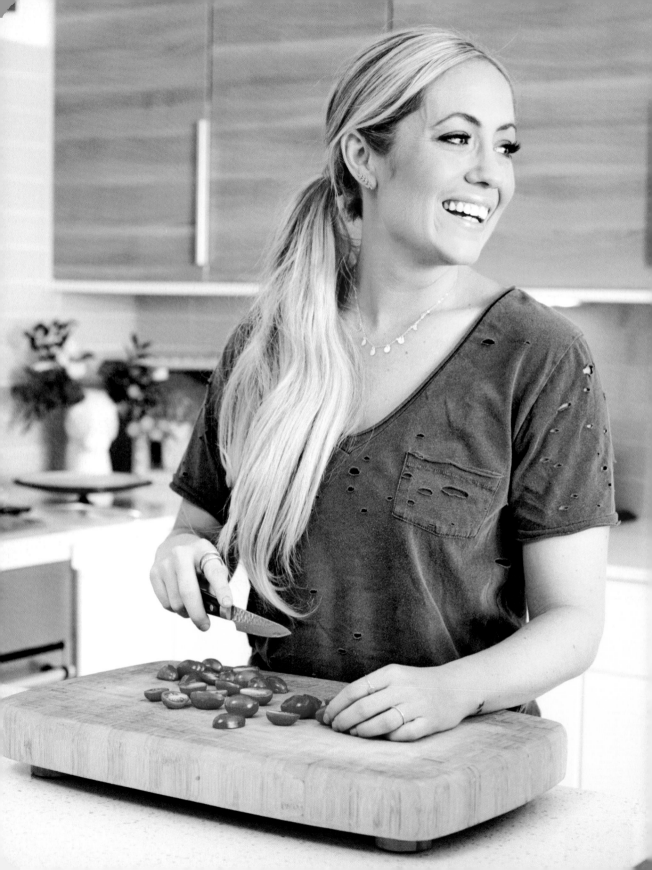

Seven

Aim True in the Kitchen:
50 RECIPES to SEDUCE YOUR INNER TOP CHEF

Now that we have some intentions set, it's time to dive in.

You may have noticed by now that my approach to health is open-minded. I have some specific universal beliefs about what's good for everyone (minimal to no dairy, easy on the wheat, eat more vegetables, cut out the processed foods), but I don't believe there is one way to eat for everyone (vegan, vegetarian, raw, Paleo, etc.). We're all unique, with different needs, tending to them as best we can.

For me, aiming true in health is listening to what my body needs and allowing others to do what serves them best. The recipes in this chapter are straightforward and accessible, and tend to be dairy-free (olive or coconut oil can be substituted for ghee/butter) and mostly gluten-free. I'm pretty sure after you try my Maple Cashew Cornflake Ice Cream, Cashew Nacho Cheese, and Butternut Squash Mac 'n' Cheese, you'll be converted. Can I get an amen?

Be creative, make substitutions—it's my wish that this book gives you permission to soar in your cooking and consuming. Listen to your body, be open to new flavors and possibilities, and eat up!

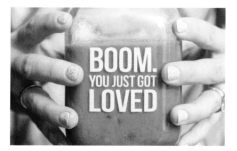

POWER SIDE KICK: VEGGIES + SIDES

MAIN ATTRACTION: ENTREES

YES, PLEASE: DESSERTS

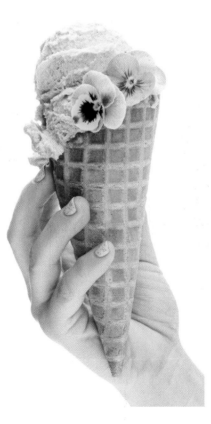

Quinoa Egg Power Bites

MAKES 12 BITES

Well, hello, little nuggets of power! These energy bites are full of flavor. They're a breeze to pull together and a great way to get some protein if you're on the go, so I constantly take them on planes (along with mini bottles of hot sauce). Guaranteed way to make the passenger next to you green with envy. Even better, take along some to share!

1 cup tricolor quinoa (see Sidebar page 153)
2 cups vegetable broth
2 tablespoons ghee or extra-virgin olive oil
3 eggs, lightly beaten
1 cucumber, shredded
½ cup pecorino cheese, shaved, or nutritional yeast
¼ cup basil, julienned
2 teaspoons cumin
1 teaspoon cayenne
2 teaspoons sea salt
12 whole pecans or walnuts (optional)
hot sauce to taste (optional)

1 Preheat the oven to 350°F.

2 Soak the quinoa for 5 minutes and drain. In a saucepan over high heat, combine the quinoa with the broth and 1 tablespoon of the ghee and bring it to a boil. Stir well, reduce the heat to low, and cook, covered, for 10 to 15 minutes, or until the quinoa is fluffy.

3 Combine the eggs, cucumber, cheese, basil, cumin, cayenne, salt, and remaining ghee in a large bowl. Stir in the quinoa.

4 Pour the mixture into a 12-cup nonstick muffin tin and top with the nuts, if desired. Bake the power bites for 20 minutes. Remove them from the tin and let cool on a rack so you don't burn your excited mouth. Douse them in hot sauce if you like an extra kick!

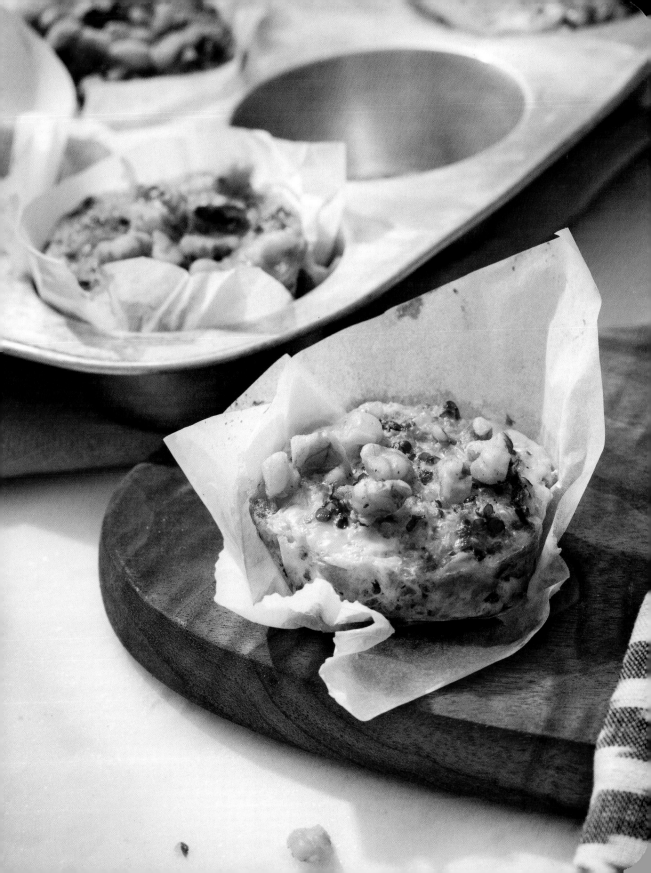

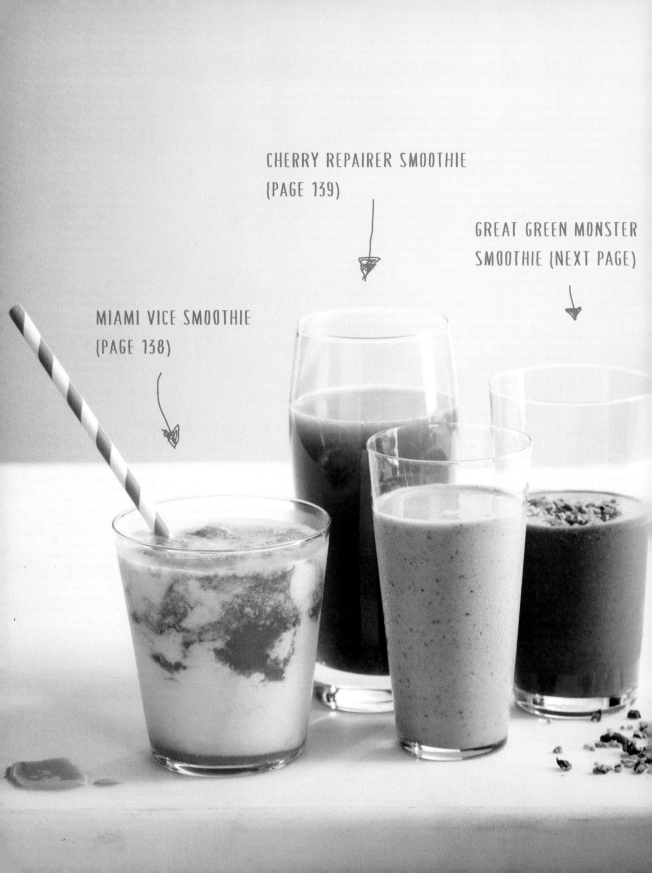

CHERRY REPAIRER SMOOTHIE
(PAGE 139)

GREAT GREEN MONSTER
SMOOTHIE (NEXT PAGE)

MIAMI VICE SMOOTHIE
(PAGE 138)

Great Green Monster Smoothies

This green mountain of goodness was inspired by a twelve-dollar smoothie I loved in Santa Monica—that was sure to break the bank. I put my taste buds to work and came up with a similar creation that made my body and wallet sing! Maca powder is a great energy lifter, cacao nibs give an antioxidant boost, and local bee pollen can help combat allergies.

1 Place the powders, spinach, mint, almonds, coconut milk, maple syrup, and 15 ice cubes into a high-powered blender and blend until smooth. Keep adding ice cubes until you've reached your desired consistency.

2 Sprinkle the cacao nibs and bee pollen on top for garnish.

¼ cup powdered greens (see Note)
1 tablespoon maca powder
2 cups raw spinach
½ cup fresh mint
10 raw almonds
1 cup coconut milk
2 tablespoons maple syrup or raw honey
15 to 20 ice cubes
1 teaspoon cacao nibs
1 teaspoon bee pollen

Note: There are many green powders on the market. I've noted some of my favorites on page 311, or feel free to replace them with extra spinach.

Miami Vice Smoothies

I had my first actual alcoholic Miami Vice (a combination strawberry daiquiri and piña colada) at a tiny bar in the Cayman Islands. It was a beautiful sunrise of colors, not to mention incredibly tasty. I figured a nonalcoholic version would bring me back to my happy beach memories with a healthy spin.

Strawberry Daiquiri

2 cups frozen
    strawberries
2 cups coconut water
½ cup lemon juice
¼ cup lime juice
1 tablespoon berry
    superfood powder
    (optional)

Piña Colada

1 cup coconut milk
2 tablespoons coconut oil
    (or coconut-flavored
    omega oil)
2 cups frozen pineapple

1   Place all the ingredients for the Strawberry Daiquiri into a high-powered blender and blend until smooth. Place in a pitcher.

2   Place all the ingredients for the Piña Colada into a high-powered blender and blend until smooth. Pour some of the Piña Colada into a glass, followed by an equal amount of the Strawberry Daiquiri. Hit it with a straw, throw on some shades, and kick your feet up.

Cherry Repairer Smoothies

I've been so smitten with cherries this season that I took the time to get to know them better. Turns out they're a fantastic way to help your muscles repair faster after workouts because they possess compounds called anthocyanins, which have antioxidant properties. I knew I had to incorporate them into my A.M. smoothie rotation, and this has become my go-to anti-inflammatory drink. You can use frozen cherries if they aren't in season.

Place all the ingredients into a high-powered blender and blend until smooth.

1 cup canned light coconut milk
½ cup unsweetened almond milk
1½ cups dark sweet cherries, pitted
¼ cup raw almonds
1 teaspoon vanilla extract
2 teaspoons maple syrup
pinch of sea salt

Ready, Set, GO! Juices

MAKES 2 SHOTS OF EACH JUICE

One of my favorite juice bars sells a set of four shots called a "Grand Slam," meant to be drunk consecutively and with gusto! It inspired me to create a stoplight of shots: red, yellow, and green, with a nice airbag chaser shot to mellow out the kick! This takes a bit of preparing, but is amazingly invigorating and a fun post-workout social experience with friends.

Airbag
½ cup cubed fresh
   pineapple
4 sprigs mint
1 lemon, cut into small
   pieces
¼ cucumber, roughly
   chopped

Yellow
1 small orange, peeled
½ yellow bell pepper,
   sliced
½-inch piece fresh
   ginger, peeled
½ lemon, cut into small
   pieces

Green
1 cup wheatgrass, or 2 cups kale or spinach
1 lemon, cut into small pieces
1-inch piece fresh ginger, peeled
¼ apple, sliced

Red
2 garlic cloves, peeled
½-inch piece fresh ginger, peeled
¼ cup diced fresh pineapple
¼ beet, diced
½-inch piece turmeric root, peeled
8 sprigs basil
3 stems cilantro
½ lemon, cut into small pieces

To Finish
manuka honey or local honey
cayenne

1 Run all the Airbag ingredients through the juicer. Pour it into shot glasses.

2 Repeat this process, first with the Yellow ingredients, then the Green, then the Red (working from lightest color to darkest, so that no juice—especially the red—can tint the batch you do next).

3 Stir about ½ teaspoon honey into each shot of red juice. Line up your juices in this order: red, yellow, green, airbag. Sprinkle a little cayenne on the red, yellow, and green juices. Pound the table to work yourself up. Drink them in order, from red to airbag. Feel the juice hit your veins, and go take on the world! This is an awesome way to energize your system and make you ready for anything.

Overnight Oats

Are you bored with breakfast but feel you possess some creative juices? Then this is the recipe for you! All you need is a mason jar, rolled oats, and a good flavor palette. I'll get you started with the recipe below, but feel free to play with your milks, yogurts, and fruits as well as different spices. Just mix it all up and let it chill overnight. Breakfast has never been easier!

½ cup rolled oats

1 cup plain coconut yogurt (see Note)

1 cup unsweetened almond milk

¼ cup chia seeds

¼ cup slivered almonds

½ cup fresh fruit such as cherries, strawberries, or mango, cut into bite-size pieces if necessary

2 teaspoons vanilla or almond extract

¼ cup unsweetened coconut flakes

1 to 2 tablespoons maple syrup

Note: Use coconut yogurt, not coconut-flavored yogurt.

Place all the ingredients into a mason jar and mix well. Refrigerate overnight, and voilà! It's ready to go. Eat immediately or enjoy on the road.

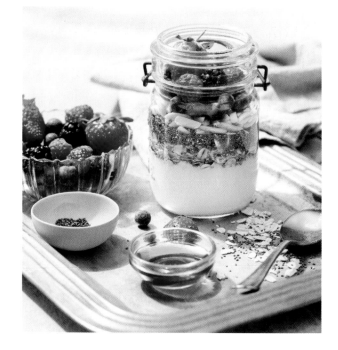

California Toast

I was terrified of avocado and its bizarre mushy consistency until I moved to the promised land of Southern California. There, those amazing fruits took on a whole new personality, as they were included in almost anything and everything you ordered. I now adore them and their health benefits—they are full of omega fatty acids. Avocado toast is one of the tastiest ways to start the day. Keep it simple, or enjoy it with a lovely sauce like my Spicy Tomato Jam (page 179).

1 Toast the bread to your liking. Take a piece of the garlic clove and rub the cut side rapidly onto the warm toast. Give each piece a solid garlic coating.

2 Divide the avocado between each piece of toast and smoosh it down with the back side of a fork (you can even get fancy and create patterns like a Zen garden). Sprinkle it with red pepper flakes, sea salt, and Spicy Tomato Jam, if desired.

2 slices gluten-free bread
1 garlic clove, halved
½ ripe avocado
1 teaspoon red pepper flakes
good pinch of sea salt
Spicy Tomato Jam (page 179; optional)

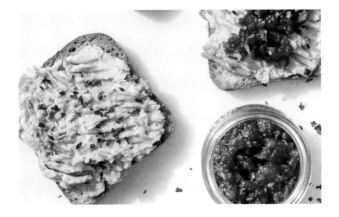

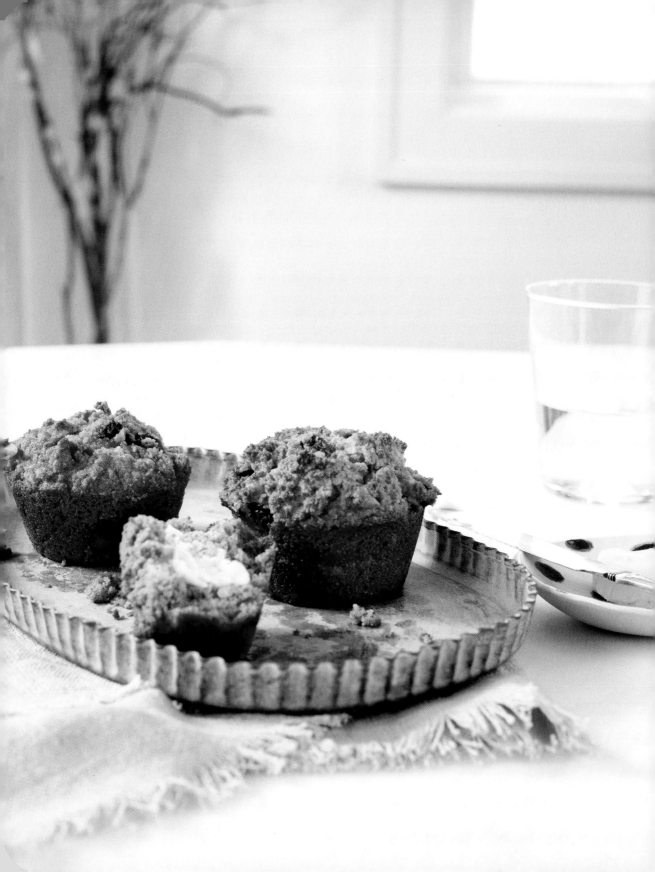

Mighty Blueberry Lemon Muffins

MAKES ABOUT 16 MUFFINS

This recipe has lived many lives. I first made it thinking it would be a dessert cake, but it turned into more of a breakfast bread. These muffins are made with juicy blueberries, tart lemon, warming almond, and coconut flour, which is chock-full of fiber, so it's a great way to fuel you up for the day and keep you full. Serve these muffins (or bread, see Note) with a delicious tea or coffee, or even use them as a healthy dessert.

1 Preheat the oven to 350°F and spray two nonstick muffin pans with coconut oil. Using a stand or hand mixer, combine all the ingredients except the blueberries and slivered almonds. Fold in the blueberries and almonds, just until combined. Pour the batter into the prepared pans, filling each cup to the top. You will not fill all the cups in the second tin.

2 Bake the muffins for 20 minutes, or until a wooden skewer inserted into the center of a muffin comes out clean. Pop the muffins out onto cooling racks, and let them rest for about 10 minutes.

¾ cup coconut flour
½ cup maple syrup
6 eggs
1 teaspoon baking soda
⅓ cup apple butter
¼ cup coconut oil
1 cup fresh ground almond butter
1½ teaspoons almond extract
zest and juice of 1 lemon
pinch of sea salt
1 pint fresh blueberries
1 cup slivered almonds

Note: To prepare this as a bread, pour the batter into a greased 9-inch loaf tin and bake for 40 minutes.

Treat Yo'self Protein Bars

MAKES 12 BARS

My doctor wants me to eat protein at every meal, but I struggle to find ways of incorporating it without feeling heavy. I'm not a fan of store-bought protein bars, because their consistency is too powdery and thick. I decided to blend my childhood desires with my protein needs to make a chewy chocolate chip bar full of protein, fiber, energy, and tasty treats.

4 eggs
1 tablespoon coconut oil
¾ cup apple butter
¼ cup maple syrup
2 teaspoons almond extract
½ cup coconut flour
½ cup vanilla protein powder
2 tablespoons ground flaxseeds
1 teaspoon sea salt
2 teaspoons cinnamon
1 cup unsweetened coconut flakes
¾ cup chocolate chips
½ cup chia seeds
1 cup slivered almonds

1. Preheat the oven to 375°F and place a silicone liner on a baking sheet. In a large bowl, whisk together the eggs, coconut oil, apple butter, maple syrup, and almond extract.

2. Slowly whisk in the coconut flour, protein powder, flaxseeds, salt, and cinnamon. Fold in the coconut flakes, chocolate chips, chia seeds, and almonds.

3. Grab about a golf-ball-size piece of dough and roll it into a narrow log shape about 3 inches long. Pat the log into a rectangular shape.

4. Arrange the bars, evenly spaced, on the prepared sheet and bake for 15 minutes. Let cool for 5 minutes.

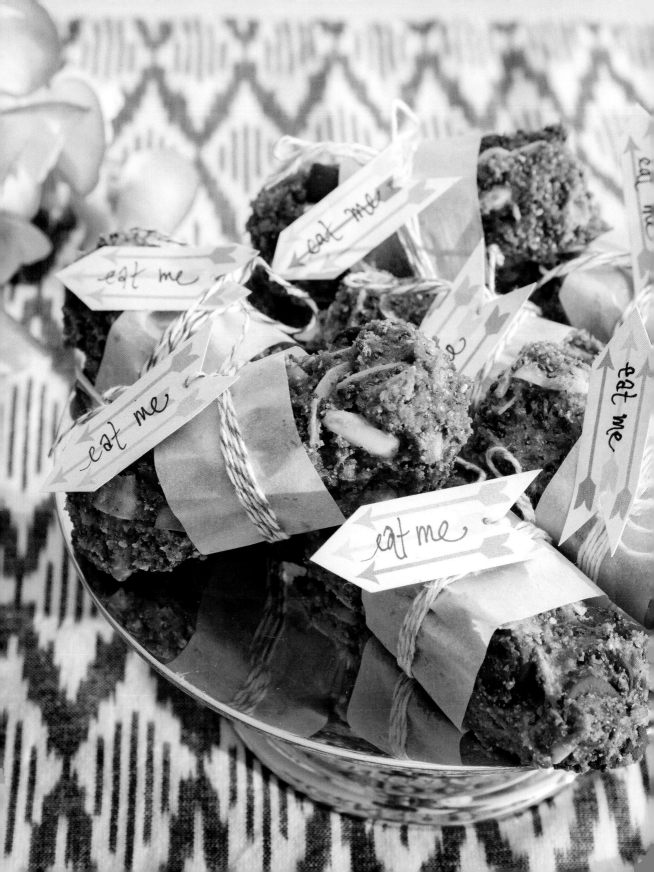

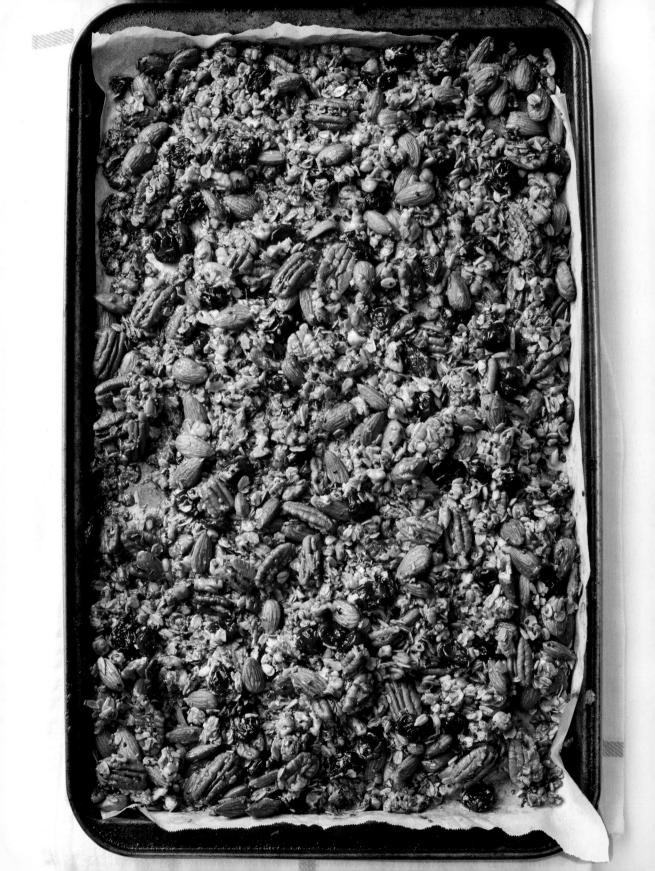

I Can't Quit You Granola

MAKES 8 CUPS

I used to make this granola weekly with my friend Julie Rhee when I lived in Venice, California. It was our take on the highly addictive granola found at our favorite restaurant, Axe. Axe has since closed down, but its epic granola will live on forever! This granola should seriously come with a warning label—forget the spoon and pack a shovel.

1. Preheat the oven to 350°F. Combine the ghee, brown sugar, and honey in a small pot and cook the mixture over low heat until the butter melts and the sugar dissolves. Stir until fully combined.

2. Spread the oats and all of the nuts and seeds on a cookie sheet lined with parchment paper. Drizzle the ghee mixture over the granola mixture and stir until all the pieces are coated with a lovely goo.

3. Bake for 10 minutes. Remove the sheet and give it a good toss with a wooden spoon, then fold the cherries into the mix. Continue baking the granola for another 8 minutes; let it cool. Break apart the pieces and store them for up to 2 weeks, although I highly doubt they will last that long.

½ cup ghee
½ cup dark brown sugar
½ cup raw honey
3 cups rolled oats
2 cups pecans
1 cup whole raw almonds
1 cup walnuts
½ cup flaxseeds
½ cup sunflower seeds
½ cup black sesame seeds
1 cup dried cherries

Secret Garden Farro Salad

MAKES 2 TO 3 SERVINGS

I've never met a farro I didn't like. The nutty Italian grain brings an instant smile to my face. It can be served warm or at room temperature. This is a refreshing salad, with flavors reminiscent of a vibrant spring garden.

4 cups chicken or
    vegetable broth
1 cup dry farro
pinch of sea salt
¼ cup walnut oil
¼ cup fig balsamic
    vinegar
juice of 1 lemon
handful flat-leaf parsley,
    roughly chopped
smoked sea salt
¼ cup dried cherries
1 cup golden cherry
    tomatoes
4 cups arugula
5 radishes, sliced
½ yellow beet, thinly
    sliced and quartered

1 Combine the broth, farro, and salt in a saucepan over high heat and bring the mixture to a boil. Reduce the heat to maintain a simmer and cook for 30 minutes, or until al dente. Drain the farro using a fine-mesh sieve and transfer it to a large bowl to cool.

2 Whisk together the oil, vinegar, lemon juice, and parsley in a medium bowl and season with smoked salt to taste. In a large serving bowl, combine the cherries, tomatoes, arugula, radishes, and beet. Stir in the cooled farro, pour the dressing over the salad, and toss to combine.

To Salt or Not to Salt

You'll notice I rarely give exact measurements of salt, but rather call for a "pinch" or salting "to taste." Salt is a very personal (and delicious) thing, but can easily be overdone. I recommend always starting on the light side and then tasting as you go. Using beautiful finishing sea salt flakes (like Maldon) is a great way to add that extra salting pop and bring out the flavor without dousing your food with sodium.

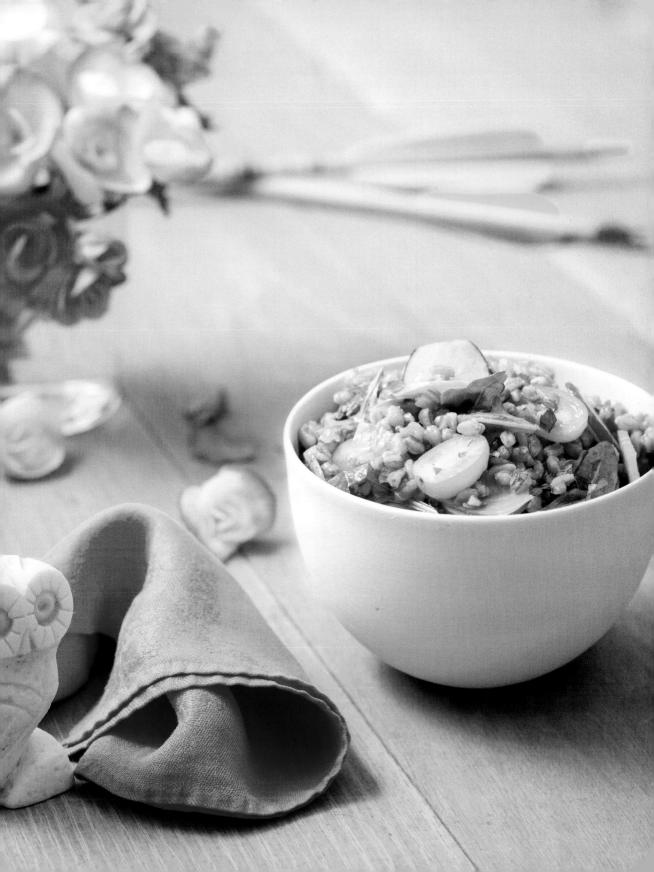

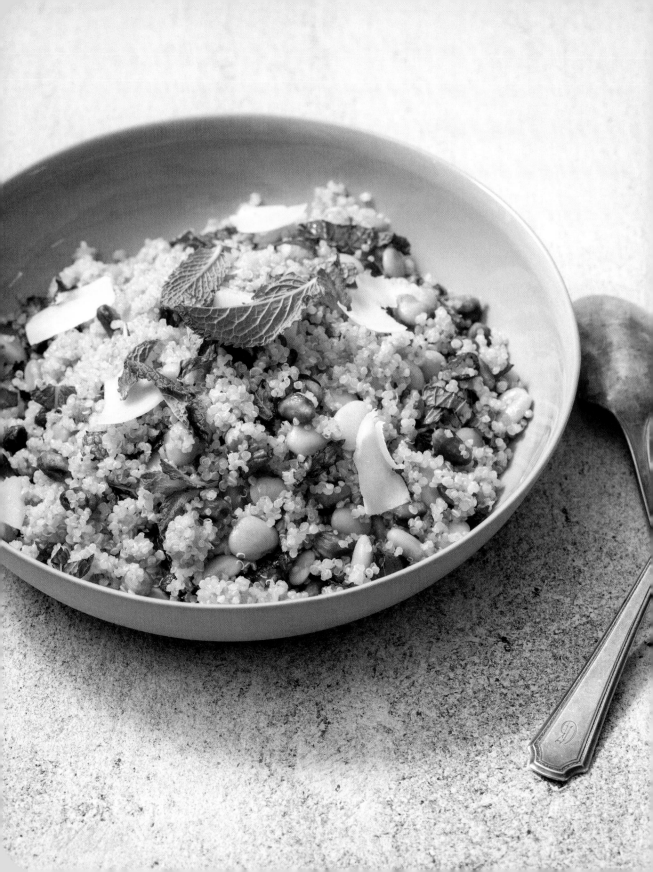

Bright Quinoa Salad

This is one of my favorite go-to salads on a warm day. Its bright flavors help to relax and cool, while the quinoa fills you up and adds protein.

1 In a large saucepan, bring the quinoa to a boil with the vegetable broth and sea salt. Stir well and reduce the heat to maintain a simmer. Stir often over the next 10 to 15 minutes, until the seeds have popped and become fluffy.

2 In a large bowl, combine the quinoa with all the remaining ingredients. Toss well and serve immediately.

Quinoa Bathtub

Quinoa is one of my favorite foods, but many people find it hard to digest. If that's true for you, try this simple trick: soak it in a bowl of water overnight or for at least an hour, and drain it in a fine-mesh strainer before cooking as directed. This soaking process removes the outer shell of phytic acid, making it easier to digest. When short on time, at least give it a good rinse or soak for 5 minutes.

2 cups white quinoa
(see Sidebar)
4 cups vegetable broth
sea salt
¼ cup shaved Parmesan
1 cup shelled pistachios
2 cups frozen fava or
lima beans, thawed
½ cup mint leaves,
roughly chopped
2 tablespoons extra-
virgin olive oil
zest of 1 lemon
juice of 2 lemons

Foraged Salad with Crispy Lemon

I first had this showstopping salad at Cochon in New Orleans. This is my interpretation, and it brings me back to my happy place every time. The soft yet bright lemon flavor comes from my favorite citrus by far, Meyer lemons. It's as if an orange and a lemon had a baby. They are seasonal, so feel free to replace them with regular lemons if need be.

2 tablespoons extra-virgin olive oil

2 fennel bulbs, fronds removed and reserved, bulbs thinly sliced

pinch of sea salt

12 ounces white mushrooms, thinly sliced

3 cups safflower oil

1 Meyer lemon, thinly sliced

Dressing and Finish

juice of 2 Meyer lemons

¼ cup extra-virgin olive oil

¼ cup champagne vinegar

2 garlic cloves, minced

2 teaspoons smoked salt

1 shallot, finely chopped

¼ cup flat-leaf parsley, chopped

¼ cup mint, chopped

1 Heat the olive oil in a large pan over medium heat, and sauté the sliced fennel, seasoned with sea salt, for 5 to 7 minutes, or until soft. Add the mushrooms and sauté for another 3 to 5 minutes until they relax and release their juices. Transfer the mixture into a bowl.

2 Heat the safflower oil over high heat and drop the lemon slices into it to fry for 10 minutes. Remove them with a slotted spoon and place them on paper towels to drain. Pat them gently and add them to the fennel and mushrooms.

3 To make the dressing, combine the lemon juice, oil, vinegar, garlic, salt, and shallot in a large bowl and mix well. Pour this over the mushroom mixture, toss well, and top off the salad with the parsley and mint. Garnish with the reserved fennel fronds. Serve immediately.

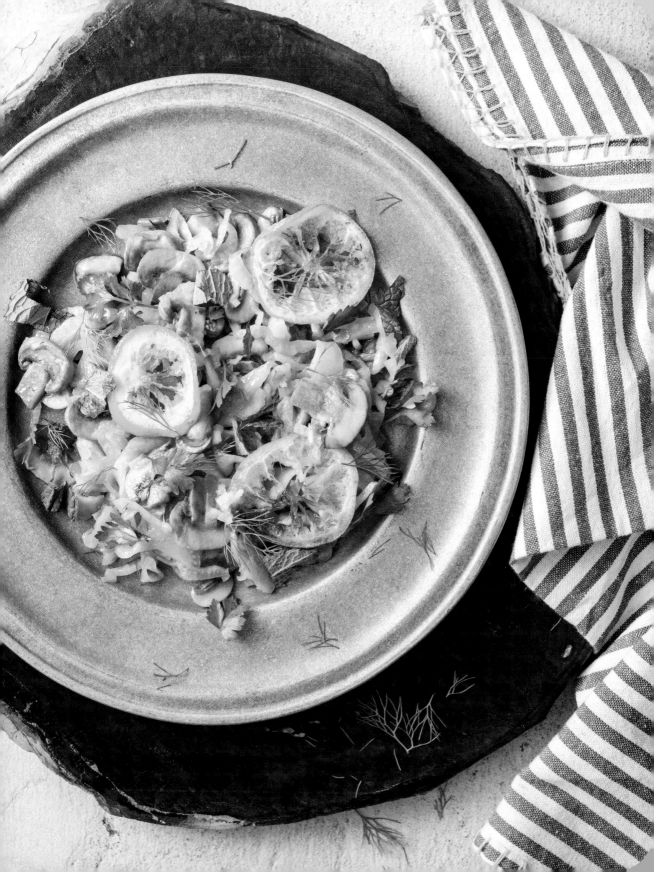

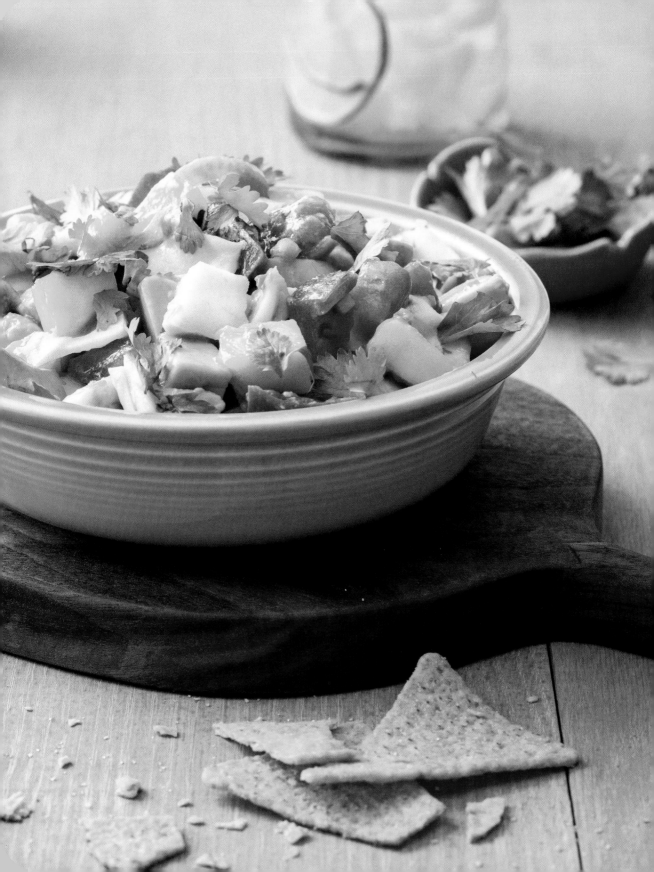

Coconut Ceviche

My beautiful friend Victoria Dodge first introduced this little cup of genius into my life. Her spin on the traditional Peruvian fish dish inspired me to attempt my own twist, and judging from the empty bowls at the dinner table, it was a success. This is a great snack, lunch, or simple way to impress your dinner guests.

1 In a small bowl, combine the red onion, vinegar, and salt; set the mixture aside to quick-pickle for 10 minutes.

2 Meanwhile, cut the coconut meat into bite-size pieces and place it in a large serving bowl. Add the avocado, mango, tomato, and jalapeño to the bowl.

3 To make the dressing, in a cup, whisk together the lime juice, oil, salt, sambal, and ginger. Pour the dressing over the salad and stir. Drain the pickled onions and add them to the bowl. Top it with the cilantro. Serve the ceviche in bowls or with tortilla chips for dipping.

Note: To open a fresh coconut, cut a small square shape at the top with a cleaver and then pry it open with a knife. Or make your life easier and ask someone behind the counter to do it for you at the store. Peel out all the coconut meat with a spoon. Don't forget to save the coconut water for drinking or smoothies!

½ red onion, thinly sliced
½ cup apple cider vinegar
1 teaspoon sea salt
1 cup fresh coconut meat, from 1 to 2 coconuts (see Note)
1 avocado, diced
½ mango, diced
1 ripe heirloom tomato, diced
½ green jalapeño, finely chopped

Dressing and Finish
juice of 2 limes
¼ cup extra-virgin olive oil
pinch of sea salt
1 tablespoon sambal oelek (see Note page 169)
½-inch piece fresh ginger, peeled and diced
leaves from 1 small bunch cilantro
tortilla chips, for serving (optional)

Kick-Ass Kale Salad

This salad was love and slobber at first Instagram picture. A friend posted a picture of herself enjoying this salad and I was the first to message for more details. It is full of nutrients (all hail kale) and provides a spectrum of colors and mini flavor bombs. Even the most committed meat eaters will devour this baby.

2 carrots, peeled and sliced

2 tablespoons agave nectar

1 tablespoon paprika

sea salt

5 tablespoons extra-virgin olive oil

1 bunch lacinato kale, roughly chopped

1 (3.5-ounce) jar capers, drained

¼ cup lemon-infused extra-virgin olive oil (see Note page 177)

1 preserved lemon, chopped (see Sidebar page 171)

¼ cup white wine vinegar

1 shallot, finely diced

½ red onion, sliced

¼ cup grated raw Parmesan

1 Preheat the oven to 450°F. Toss the carrots with the agave, paprika, 1 tablespoon sea salt, and 2 tablespoons of the olive oil. Spread the mixture on a cookie sheet and roast for 30 minutes.

2 Massage the chopped kale with 2 tablespoons of the olive oil and a dusting of sea salt. Set it aside. (It's good to let the kale sit in the oil for 10 to 15 minutes before serving.)

3 Warm the remaining 1 tablespoon olive oil in a sauté pan over medium-high heat. Add the capers and dust them lightly with sea salt. Fry, stirring often, for about 5 minutes.

4 In a bowl, whisk together the lemon olive oil, preserved lemon, vinegar, shallot, and salt to taste. Place the kale in a serving bowl and add the roasted carrots, fried capers, and sliced onion; toss to mix. Top the salad with the dressing, transfer it to individual salad bowls, and sprinkle with the raw Parm.

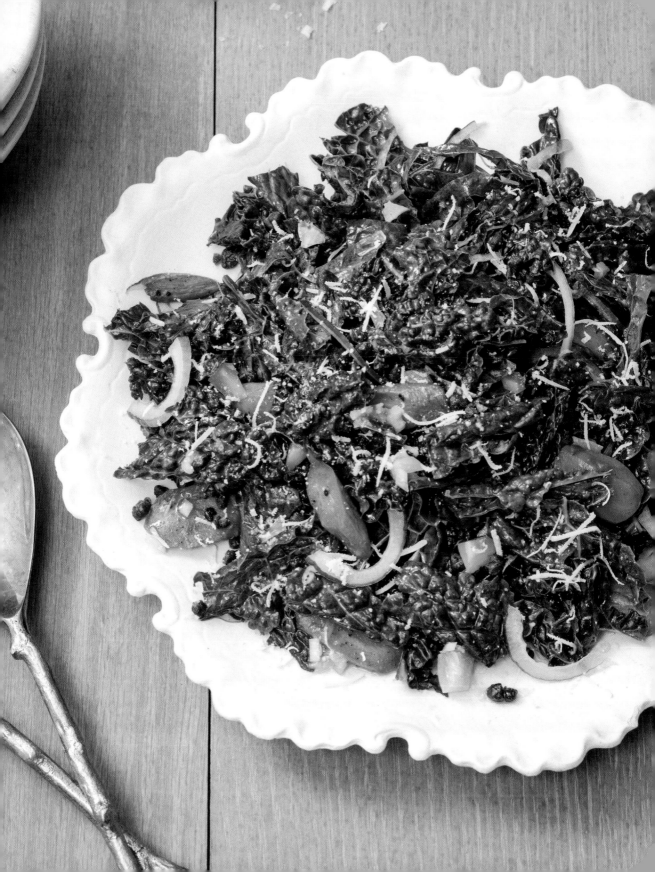

Red Quinoa Apricot Salad

MAKES 4 SERVINGS

Quinoa is a staple in my diet, so I'm always on a mission to find new creative ways to make it shine. The sweetness of apricot and richness of sweet potato make this meal awesome.

Dressing

½ cup extra-virgin olive oil

½ cup apple cider vinegar

juice of ½ Meyer or small regular lemon

2 teaspoons maple syrup

3 dried apricots

1 tablespoon whole-grain Dijon mustard

1 teaspoon sea salt

Salad

2 cups cherry tomatoes, quartered

2 tablespoons white wine vinegar

2 teaspoons garlic powder

5 tablespoons extra-virgin olive oil

1 cup red quinoa (see Sidebar page 153)

1 sweet potato, cubed

1 shallot, diced

1 teaspoon red pepper flakes

sea salt

2 cups vegetable broth

3 spring onions, white and green parts thinly sliced

10 dried apricots, thinly sliced

large sprig of basil, julienned

roughly 5 cups wild arugula

goat cheese to taste (optional)

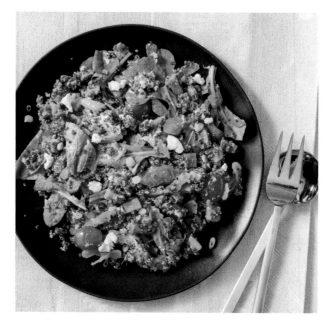

1 Place all of the dressing ingredients into a blender and puree until smooth. It may take a few rounds to fully blend the apricots. Set aside.

2 In a bowl, combine the cherry tomatoes, vinegar, and garlic powder with 3 tablespoons of the oil. Stir well and set aside to marinate for 20 minutes. Place the quinoa in a bowl with enough water to cover and allow it to soak for at least 5 minutes.

3 Heat 1 tablespoon of the oil in a large sauté pan over medium-low. Sauté the sweet potato and shallot with the red pepper flakes and a pinch of salt for 10 to 15 minutes, or until the potato is soft.

4 Drain the quinoa and place it in a large saucepan with the broth, the remaining olive oil, and a pinch of salt. Bring the mixture to a boil and stir well. Reduce the heat to low and cook the quinoa, covered, for 10 to 15 minutes, or until it is fluffy. Let it cool slightly.

5 Place the spring onions, apricots, and basil in a large serving bowl. Add the arugula, quinoa, and dressing. Gently fold the salad together. Add small blots of cheese, if desired.

Watermelon and Roasted Tomato Gazpacho

MAKES 4 SERVINGS

My favorite gazpacho hails from Le Pain Quotidien. I've begged and begged for the recipe without success, so I decided to take the matter into my own hands. Problem was, I got distracted by a watermelon. So I threw it into the mix, and my new favorite gazpacho was born. This will woo over warm-soup lovers everywhere.

2 cups cherry tomatoes, halved

¼ cup extra-virgin olive oil, plus more for roasting

2 teaspoons sea salt

2 teaspoons red pepper flakes

2 cups watermelon

5 radishes, diced

1 mango, diced

1 Preheat the oven to 400°F.

2 Place the tomatoes on a cookie sheet and dose them with a glug of olive oil. Sprinkle them evenly with the sea salt and red pepper flakes. Mix well and roast for 25 to 30 minutes.

3 Transfer the tomatoes to a blender. Add the watermelon and quick-pulse twice for a few seconds each time to keep a chunky consistency or longer for smooth.

4 Pour the gazpacho into serving bowls and top it with radishes and mango.

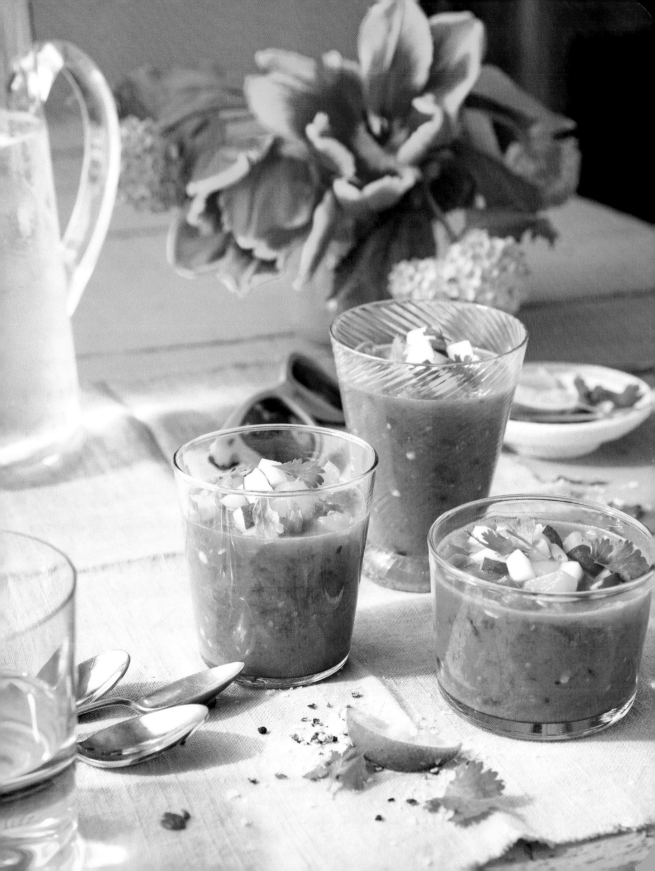

Miang Kham (Swiss Chard Wraps)

These little pockets of joy are traditional snack food in Thailand and one of my all-time favorite things to prepare. I normally enjoy these with my girlfriends and several bottles of wine. I prep all the ingredients and turn us into an assembly line until every flavorful morsel is wrapped up in its green leaf burrito. The result? A happy dance in your mouth. Make a ton—these are poppable and go fast!

½ cup unsweetened coconut flakes

1 stalk lemongrass, sliced

2 tablespoons grated fresh ginger

½ cup hot water

1 tablespoon fish sauce

½ cup tamarind paste or quince paste

½ cup coconut or brown sugar

1 tablespoon coconut oil

10 shrimp, cooked and cut into thirds

1 teaspoon seasoned or spicy salt

1 bunch Swiss chard, cleaned and torn to hand-size pieces

3 shallots, slivered

2-inch piece fresh ginger, slivered

2 to 3 jalapeño and/or red chile peppers, thinly sliced

½ cup peanuts

3 to 4 limes, thinly sliced and cut into small wedges

1 In a sauté pan over medium heat, toast the coconut flakes for 2 to 3 minutes, or until they are golden brown (watch closely, they burn fast). Transfer them to a bowl.

2 Add the lemongrass and grated ginger to the sauté pan and dry toast them for 2 minutes. Add the hot water, fish sauce, tamarind paste, and sugar and stir until combined. Reduce the heat to low and cook for 5 minutes. Stir in 1 tablespoon of the toasted coconut flakes, transfer the sauce to a bowl, and set it aside.

Bring the heat back up to medium-high and melt the coconut oil in the sauté pan. Add the shrimp and sprinkle them with the seasoned salt. Cook for 2 to 3 minutes, or until they are curled and pink. Chop them into small pieces.

Arrange all the ingredients within reach in this order: chard, shallots, ginger, jalapeños, the remaining toasted coconut, shrimp, peanuts, sauce, and lime wedges. Start with a piece of chard and add a pinch each of shallots and ginger, 1 to 2 pieces of the jalapeños, a pinch of toasted coconut, a few bits of shrimp, 1 to 2 peanuts, a drizzle of sauce, and the juice from a lime wedge. Roll it up (don't try to make them pretty, this is street food!) and pop it into your mouth!

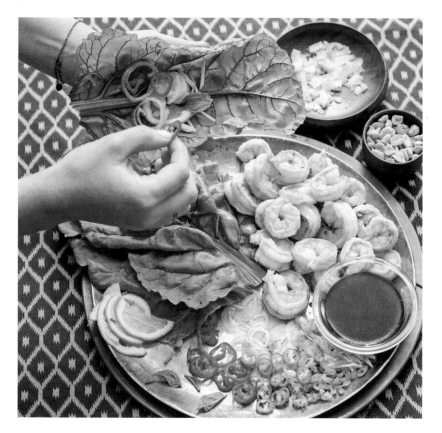

Zucchini Pasta with Almond Basil Pesto

MAKES 2 TO 4 SERVINGS

Raw cuisine isn't always my favorite (my digestion has seen better days), but I've always been impressed with veggie pasta. It's a sponge for flavor and the perfect canvas for sauce. I took a spin on the classic basil pesto by replacing pine nuts with almonds. The result is a simple, fast, refreshing lunch.

2 zucchini

¼ cup raw almonds

2 large handfuls fresh basil

¼ cup extra-virgin olive oil

¼ cup grated pecorino cheese

2 garlic cloves, peeled

2 teaspoons pink salt

1 cup cherry tomatoes, halved

1. Spiralize or peel the zucchini into noodle-like ribbons. Pat them with paper towels to remove excess liquid.

2. Place the almonds, basil, oil, pecorino, garlic, and salt into a food processor and blend until the pesto is the desired consistency (I like a chunky texture). Gently fold the pesto into the zucchini noodles and toss with the cherry tomatoes.

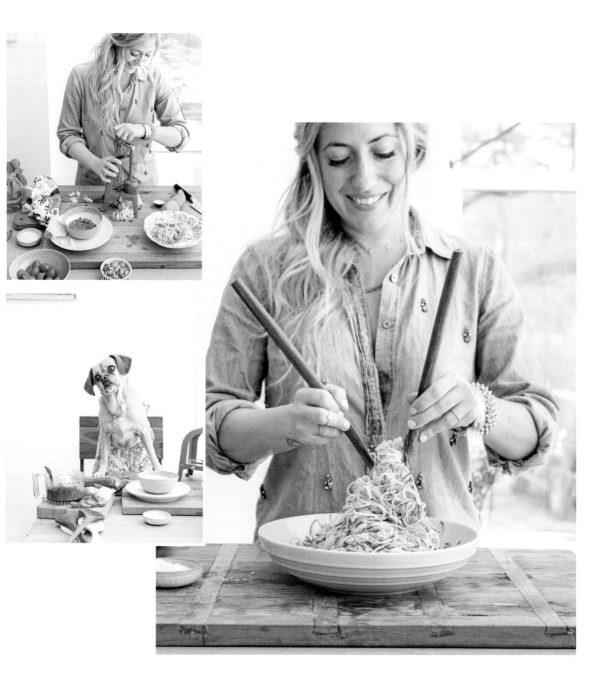

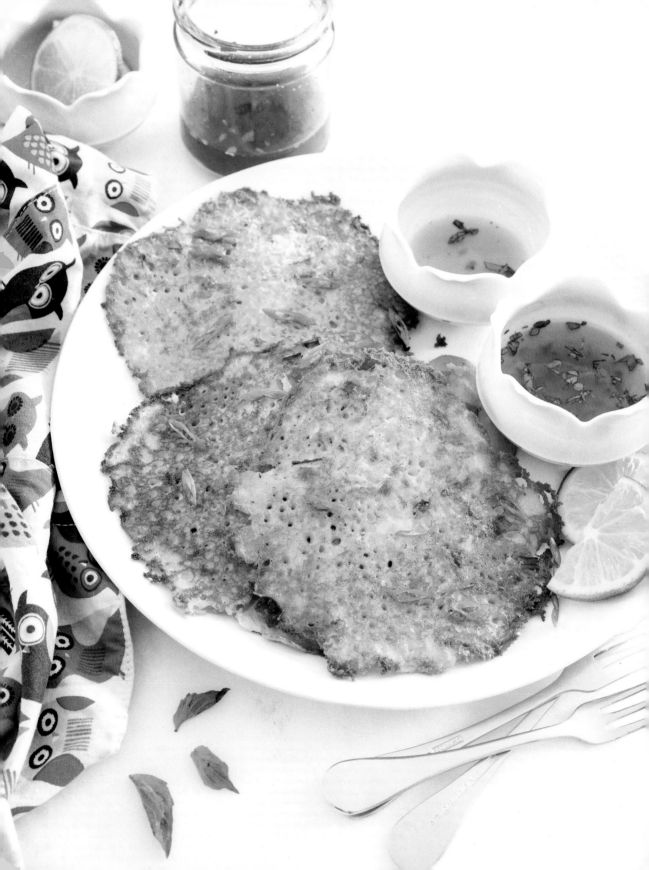

Kimchi Pancakes

My niece and nephew both hail from Korea, and this recipe is an ode to their heritage. Kimchi is a classic fermented vegetable dish, often made with cabbage, that does wonders for your digestive system and taste buds. These pancakes are a great appetizer or casual lunch. Just be sure to make plenty—they tend to get scooped up before you're even done!

1 Beat the eggs lightly in a large bowl. Slowly whisk in the rice flour, beer, tamari, kimchi juice, and sesame oil. Fold in the scallions and kimchi. Season with salt.

2 Warm 1 tablespoon of the coconut oil in a large frying pan over medium heat. Pour ½ cup of the batter into the pan. Let the pancake fry for 2 to 3 minutes per side. Repeat until all of your pancakes are made. Add more coconut oil when necessary.

3 Whisk together the dressing ingredients and dip your pancakes generously!

Note: Sambal oelek is an Indonesian chile paste that might remind you a bit of sriracha. You can find it in Asian markets, or in the Asian section of most grocery stores.

Kimchi Pancakes

2 eggs
1 cup brown rice flour
1 cup pale beer
1 tablespoon tamari
1 cup kimchi, plus a good splash of the juice
2 tablespoons toasted sesame oil
2 bunches scallions, white and green parts roughly chopped
pinch of sea salt
4 to 5 tablespoons coconut oil

Dressing

juice of 1 lime
2 tablespoons fish sauce
2 tablespoons chopped cilantro
1 tablespoon sambal oelek (see Note)
splash of kimchi juice

Quinoa Kale Tabbouleh

Tabbouleh can be phenomenal. This recipe is high in flavor and nutrition, replacing bulgur wheat with gluten-free and protein-packed quinoa. Dig in!

1 cup white quinoa, soaked for 15 to 20 minutes and drained (see Sidebar page 153)

2 cups veggie broth

1 tablespoon ghee

1 teaspoon sea salt

¼ cup extra-virgin olive oil

juice of 2 lemons

1 preserved lemon, diced (see next page)

1 cup cherry tomatoes, quartered

1 English cucumber, diced

¼ cup curly parsley, cut into chiffonade

7 scallions, slivered

¼ cup basil, cut into chiffonade

¼ cup mint, cut into chiffonade

2 tablespoons tarragon, chopped

2 cups lacinato kale, cut into chiffonade

1 In a large saucepan, bring the quinoa, veggie broth, ghee, and sea salt to a boil. Stir well, reduce the heat to low, and cover. Cook for 15 minutes, or until fluffy.

2 In a small bowl, whisk together the olive oil, lemon juice, and preserved lemon and set aside.

3 Combine the cooked quinoa with the remaining ingredients, pour the dressing over all, and mix well.

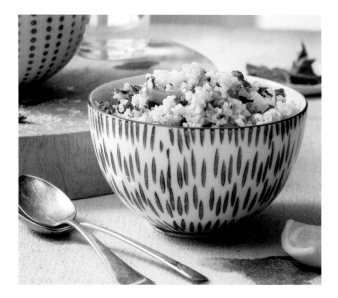

Preserved Lemons

I haven't met a lemon I haven't loved, but when they're preserved? They melt in your mouth, and they're gorgeous on top of grilled fish or whisked into a dressing. You can buy them at higher-end grocery stores or skip the price tag and make your own!

5 to 6 lemons (or whatever will fit in your large mason jar)
3 cups hot water
½ cup sugar (I use coconut sugar)
¼ cup sea salt
2 cloves

Boil the lemons for 10 minutes and let them cool. Score each one lengthwise four times. In a bowl, mix the hot water, sugar, salt, and cloves. Place the lemons in a large mason jar and pour in enough of the water mixture to cover. Let them sit for 3 to 4 weeks in the refrigerator before using.

Whole Foods Parking Lot Sammy

MAKES 1 SANDWICH

If Whole Foods had a VIP program I would be the president. I spend almost every day in that store when I'm home and have made friends with most of the people who work there. My buddy Ryan is my favorite, and he once jokingly told me about his favorite midnight snack sandwich as he brought my groceries to my car. It's the perfect blend of sweet and savory, with a nice bite to it, and it's now my favorite sandwich to pack when I travel. Thanks, Ryan!

2 tablespoons almond butter or honey-roasted peanut butter

2 slices gluten-free bread, toasted

2 teaspoons Spicy Sriracha (page 180)

5 leaves basil

1 Spread the nut butter on both sides of the bread. Add a layer of sriracha to one piece of bread and top it with an even pile of basil.

2 Assemble the sandwich, cut it in half, and let your taste buds smile.

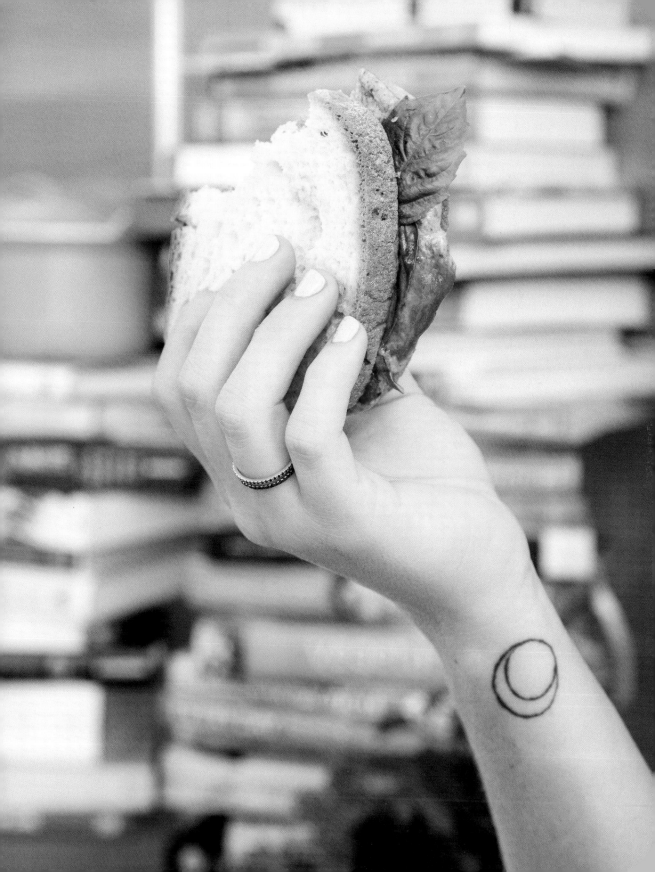

Not Your Childhood SpaghettiOs

MAKES 3 TO 4 SERVINGS

SpaghettiOs was my favorite food growing up. I now think about the processed can of suspicious noodles and quiver, yet release a sigh for the good old days. Determined to not let those little inner tubes of joy be deflated, I headed to the kitchen, armed with organic ingredients. The resulting recipe will keep every child (and adult) on cloud nine. Seriously, go make this right now. You'll be so happy.

1 bunch carrots
1 cup unsweetened
   almond milk
½ cup nutritional yeast
1 tablespoon ghee
5 spring onions, diced
1 (28-ounce) can
   crushed San Marzano
   tomatoes
2 tablespoons tomato
   paste
1 (12-ounce) bag anelletti
   noodles
sea salt

1 Juice the carrots and set the juice aside. Place the almond milk and the nutritional yeast into a blender and blend for 20 seconds. Set aside.

2 Heat the ghee in a frying pan over medium heat and sauté the spring onions for 5 minutes. Add the tomatoes, carrot juice, and tomato paste and stir well; adjust the heat to maintain a simmer and cook for another 5 minutes. Add the almond milk mixture and simmer for another 5 to 10 minutes.

3 Prepare the noodles according to the package directions and drain them.

4 Season the sauce with salt to taste and serve it over the noodles. Remember, you want an almost soupy consistency, so pour heavy!

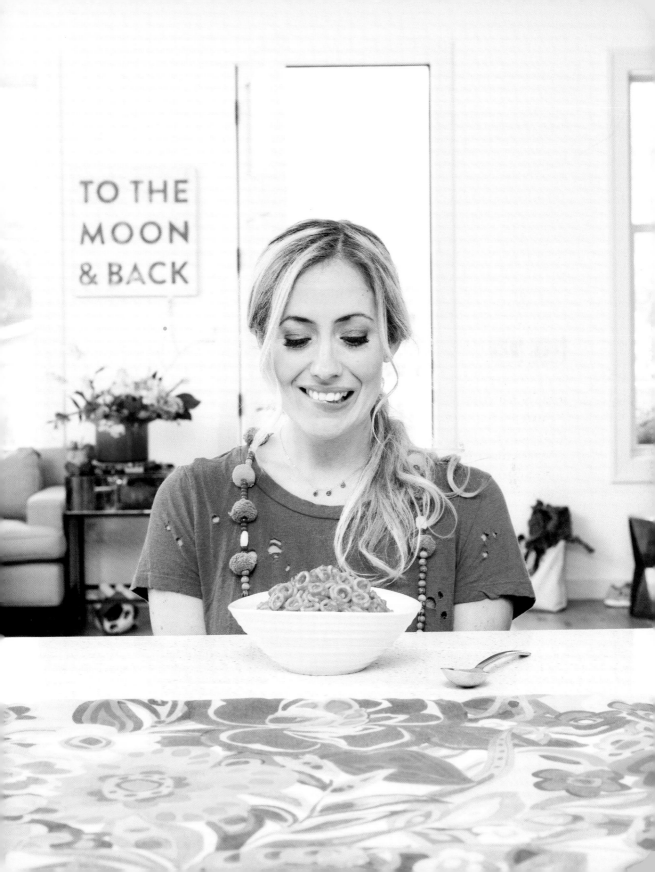

Vegan Ranch

MAKES 1 CUP

Ranch dressing is just one of those things that you hate to admit you love. This creamy dressing is a classic guilty pleasure. My lackluster affair with dairy led me to whipping up a simple dairy-free version. Go crazy with your fresh herbs (see Sidebar page 211)—the choices below are just a suggestion. This dressing pairs perfectly with the Crudités Platter (page 186) or works when you want to dunk your pizza. That's right, I learned so much in college . . .

1 cup soy-free vegan
　mayo
2 tablespoons
　unsweetened almond
　milk
1 tablespoon sweet
　onion, diced
1 small garlic clove
1 teaspoon sea salt
1 teaspoon chopped
　chives
1 teaspoon chopped
　fresh rosemary
1 teaspoon chopped
　fresh thyme
1 teaspoon chopped
　fresh sage
1 teaspoon chopped
　fresh basil

1 Place the mayo, almond milk, onion, garlic, and salt into a blender and puree until smooth. Fold in all the herbs. (If you're not a purist who likes your ranch to be white flecked with green, you can go ahead and blend everything all at once.)

2 Store in the refrigerator for up to a week.

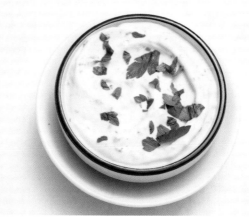

Best Hummus Ever

MAKES 3 CUPS

Hummus can either blow your mind or make you cry tears of boredom. I've been known to have quite a love affair with a good hummus, and this one will make you want to put a ring on it. The secret ingredient? *Umeboshi* (pickled plum) paste. This can be found in the Asian aisle of most markets. Pair this with the Crudités Platter (page 186) or mix it into a fresh hot bowl of quinoa. Or just eat it with a spoon. I won't tell.

1. Place all the ingredients into a blender and blend until smooth.

2. Store in the refrigerator for up to a week.

Note: If you don't have lemon-infused extra-virgin olive oil on hand, use ⅔ cup extra-virgin olive oil and the juice of three lemons instead of two.

2 (15-ounce) cans garbanzo beans, well rinsed and drained
⅓ cup lemon-infused extra-virgin olive oil (see Note)
⅓ cup extra-virgin olive oil
3 tablespoons tahini
juice of 2 lemons
2 garlic cloves, peeled
2 teaspoons cumin
1 teaspoon cayenne
1 teaspoon pink sea salt
¾ cup pickled plum (*umeboshi*) paste

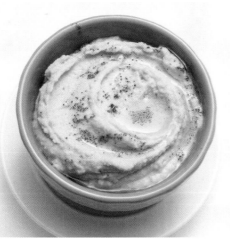

Cashew Nacho Cheese

Vegan cheese is notoriously not cheesy. Basically, it's pretty bad—it makes me long for that bloated "I'll regret this later" feeling I get from eating the real deal. The genius Ann Gentry, founder of Real Food Daily in Santa Monica, nailed it with her cashew cheese, which she would generously drizzle over nachos. It was love at first taste, and this is my take on (and ode to) her fantastic creation. I even served this to my Nebraska-born and -raised father, and he had no clue. Bam!

1 cup raw cashews, soaked for at least 2 hours or overnight
1 cup nutritional yeast
¼ sweet onion, diced
2 garlic cloves, chopped
1 tablespoon Dijon mustard
1 teaspoon cayenne
3½ cups plain unsweetened almond milk
1 cup non-GMO cornstarch
½ cup sunflower oil
¼ cup white miso
juice of 1 lemon
sea salt to taste

1. Place all the ingredients into a blender and blend until smooth, 1 to 2 minutes.

2. Transfer the mixture to a large pot and heat it over medium-low heat, whisking, until it is fully warmed.

3. Store the sauce in the refrigerator for up to a week or freeze for future use.

Spicy Tomato Jam

My dear friend Lauren Haas of Haas Holistic inspired this recipe. This delicious condiment gives you the best of the savory and sweet worlds. It'll make friends with any potato it meets (it's a fantastic dip for homemade fries). Serve it on top of grilled fish or meat, roasted vegetables, and even my California Toast (page 143).

1 Preheat the oven to 350°F. In a bowl, gently combine the tomatoes with 1 tablespoon of the coconut oil and salt and pepper to taste. Arrange them on a baking sheet and roast for 40 minutes. Set them aside.

2 Melt the remaining 2 tablespoons coconut oil over medium heat in a large, wide saucepan. Sauté the shallots and garlic for 5 minutes. Deglaze the pan with a splash of apple cider vinegar, cooking for 1 minute while scraping the bottom of the pan to incorporate any browned bits. Add the roasted tomatoes and the pepper flakes, cumin, coconut milk, lemon zest, and brown sugar. Season with salt and pepper.

3 Sauté for 20 minutes, stirring often and breaking up the tomatoes with a wooden spoon. Stir in the ginger and continue cooking for 5 minutes. Store the jam in the refrigerator for up to 2 weeks.

6 Roma tomatoes, halved
3 tablespoons coconut oil
sea salt and white pepper
2 shallots, minced
3 garlic cloves, minced
apple cider vinegar
1 teaspoon red pepper flakes
1 teaspoon cumin
½ cup coconut milk
zest of 1 lemon
½ cup dark brown sugar
1 tablespoon minced fresh ginger

Spicy Sriracha

I'm a bona fide hot sauce addict. I'm not a glutton for punishment or burned taste buds, but I do like a good kick in the pants from a secret sauce. Sriracha is a staple in our household, and this batch is clean and preservative-free. You'll also get mad brownie points for saying you make your own sriracha. And if you can only find green chile peppers, it will be just as great.

1 pound red chile peppers (ideally fresno or jalapeño), chopped

1 cup garlic cloves, chopped

½ cup apple cider vinegar

½ cup rice wine vinegar

½ cup water

¼ cup coconut sugar

pinch of smoked salt

1 tablespoon arrowroot starch

2 tablespoons fish sauce

1 Combine the peppers and garlic with the vinegars and water in a large pot over high heat; bring the mixture to a boil and cook for 10 minutes. Stir in the sugar and salt, and continue cooking for another 10 minutes.

2 Transfer the mixture to a blender and blend to your preferred level of smoothness. (I prefer to keep the sauce slightly chunky.)

3 Return the sauce to the pot and reduce the heat. Stir in the arrowroot starch to thicken; simmer for 5 minutes. Remove the pot from the heat and stir in the fish sauce. Store in the refrigerator for 3 to 6 months.

"Whip It Good" Dairy-Free Topping

Ah, Cool Whip. A mysterious concoction of chemicals that creates the most epic texture ever. As a child, I remember thinking dipping strawberries in Cool Whip was a healthy treat. I love the idea behind this classic dessert spread, sans all the unnatural ingredients. This version is simple, healthy, natural, and really, really delicious.

Whip the coconut milk, vanilla extract, raw honey, and cinnamon in a KitchenAid mixer or with a hand mixer until it begins to thicken, or for 1 minute. Store in the refrigerator for 3 to 4 days.

solid part from 1 cold (13.5-ounce) can full-fat coconut milk

2 teaspoons vanilla extract

2 tablespoons raw honey

2 teaspoons cinnamon

Roasted Sweet Roots

Roasted root vegetables = heaven. Carrots release an almost naughty sweetness when they're roasted. All they need is a pinch of seasoning love, and this side dish easily holds its weight in the spotlight.

1 bunch carrots (I like to use a mix of colors)
1 tablespoon extra-virgin olive oil
1½ tablespoons smoked paprika
sea salt
2 tablespoons maple syrup

1 Preheat the oven to 400°F. Toss the carrots with the olive oil, paprika, sea salt to taste, and 1 tablespoon of the maple syrup. Spread them evenly on a roasting pan.

2 Roast the carrots for 45 minutes, or until they begin to brown.

3 Drizzle them with the remaining maple syrup and serve.

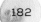

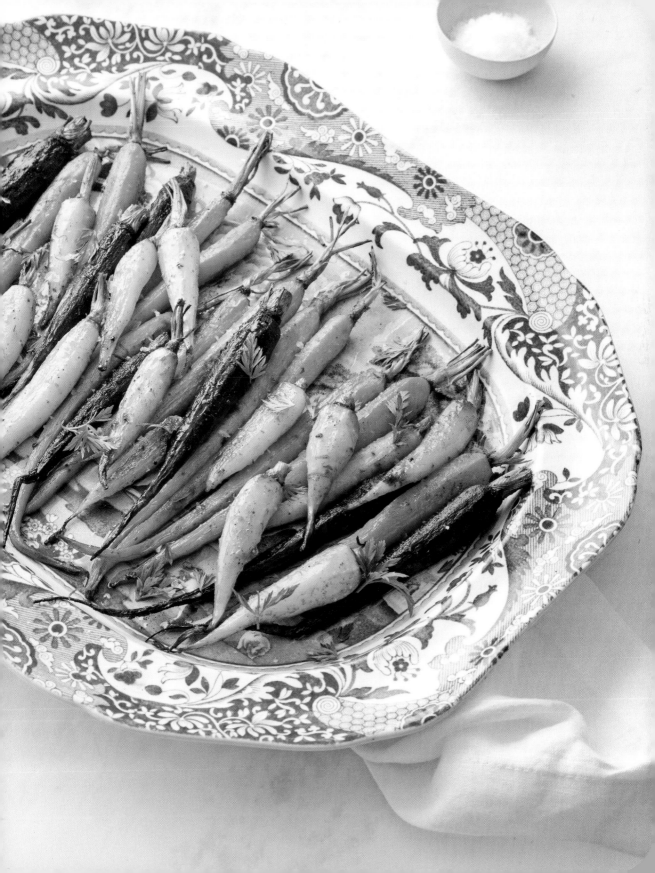

Korean Street Corn

It might be the Kansas girl in me, but I absolutely adore a grilled ear of fresh sweet corn. It's guaranteed to make you floss for hours, but worth every bite. I took my beloved corn and threw an Asian street food spin on it to give it a little pep. Awesome, messy eat-with-your-hands food!

Nom-Nom Sauce

1 tablespoon Spicy
   Sriracha (page 180) or
   gochujang (Korean hot
   pepper paste)
juice of ½ lime
2 tablespoons soy-free
   vegan mayo
2 teaspoons sea salt
1 teaspoon black pepper
1 tablespoon chopped
   chives
1 tablespoon white miso
2 teaspoons chili powder

Grilled Corn

4 ears corn, shucked and
   silks removed
2 tablespoons coconut oil
chopped cilantro, to
   garnish
chili powder, to garnish

1. Heat your grill to high or heat a grill pan over high heat.

2. Mix all the sauce ingredients together in a small bowl and set it aside.

3. Rub the ears of corn evenly with coconut oil and place them on the grill. Grill each side for about 2 minutes, or until they begin to char.

4. Drizzle sauce on each ear of grilled corn and then top with a sprinkling of cilantro and a dusting of chili powder.

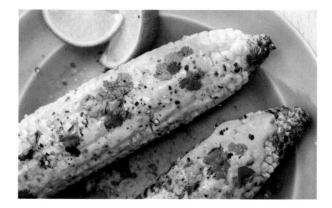

Coconut Creamed Spinach

MAKES 2 TO 4 SERVINGS

Creamed spinach was one of my childhood favorites, but as I grew up, my digestive system vetoed the cream. This recipe is a hybrid—classic creamed spinach that gives a nod to Indian cuisine. I've replaced the cream with coconut milk and experience that same bliss that I did as a young one piling spinach onto my plate.

1 Melt the ghee in a large sauté pan over medium heat. Add the red pepper flakes, a teaspoon of salt, and pepper to taste. Add the onion and cook until it caramelizes, 8 to 10 minutes.

2 Add the spinach, season with additional salt to taste, and sauté until the leaves are fully wilted. Add the coconut milk and cook for about 15 minutes to reduce the liquid.

2 to 3 tablespoons ghee
1 teaspoon red pepper flakes
pink salt
cracked black pepper
½ sweet onion, diced
6 cups spinach leaves
1 cup canned light coconut milk

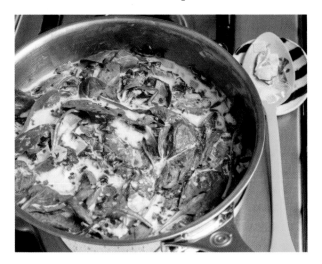

Crudités Platter

This is the perfect dish to make for a special dinner for two or a starter at a dinner party. Choose the freshest vegetables available and wash them well.

Any combination of

celery stalks

zucchinis, sliced
    lengthwise

cucumbers, sliced
    lengthwise

asparagus spears

radishes, halved

bell peppers, sliced

mini sweet peppers

cherry tomatoes, halved

multicolored carrots,
    peeled and cut into
    sticks if large

yellow beets, sliced

cauliflower, trimmed
    into small florets

broccoli, trimmed into
    small florets

Arrange the crudités artistically in a large bowl set on a base of ice. Serve with dips such as Vegan Ranch (page 176) and Best Hummus Ever (page 177).

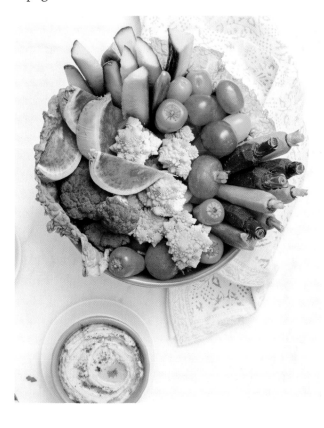

Coconut Rice

I remember the first time a girlfriend made me coconut rice. I nearly died and went to heaven right at the dinner table. Cooking with coconut milk gives this rice an amazing creamy consistency. It is delicious on its own or as a special foundation for any meal. This is the basic recipe, but feel free to get creative and add fresh herbs or spices to your liking!

1 Toast the coconut in a dry skillet over medium heat for 3 minutes or until slightly golden. (Watch closely, it burns fast!) Set it aside.

2 Add the rice, coconut milk and water, salt, and olive oil to a medium saucepan and bring the mixture to a boil over high heat. Stir well, reduce the heat to low, and cook the rice, covered, for 20 minutes, checking occasionally to mix well.

3 Serve the rice with toasted coconut flakes and scallion as garnish.

½ cup coconut flakes
1 cup jasmine rice
1 (13.5-ounce) can light coconut milk
2 cups coconut water
pinch of sea salt
splash of extra-virgin olive oil
2 scallions, greens slivered

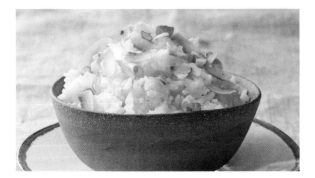

Flounder with Bourbon-Roasted Cherries and Plums

MAKES 2 SERVINGS

When in doubt, add bourbon. It might be my Charleston influence, but cooking with bourbon always seems like a good idea. In this recipe, I've used it to get cherries nice and drunk. The resulting sassy, full-bodied sauce is a great topping for this roasted fish and would do wonders over grilled red meat too.

Sauce

20 red cherries, pitted

2 black plums, pitted and diced

1 tablespoon fig balsamic vinegar

1 shallot, diced

1 teaspoon raw sugar

smoked salt

¼ cup bourbon

Fish

2 (8-ounce) fillets of flounder

sea salt

black pepper

2 tablespoons extra-virgin olive oil, plus more for drizzling

2 cups curly kale, chopped

10 yellow cherry tomatoes, halved

Coconut Rice (page 187; optional)

1. Preheat the oven to 400°F.

2. To prepare the sauce, mix the cherries, plums, vinegar, shallot, sugar, and salt in an oven-safe pan. Roast for 10 to 15 minutes. Stir in the bourbon and roast for another 5 minutes. Remove the sauce from the oven and keep it warm; leave the oven on.

3. Place the fish on an oiled baking sheet. Sprinkle it with salt and pepper to taste and drizzle it with olive oil. Roast for about 10 minutes, or until cooked through. Set aside.

4. In a frying pan, heat 2 tablespoons olive oil over medium heat and lightly sauté the

kale; season it with salt to taste. Add the kale and tomatoes to the cherry sauce.

5 Drizzle a bit of the cherry bourbon sauce on the base of the plate. Place the fish next and cover it with sauce, including some of the cherries. Serve rice on the side, if desired.

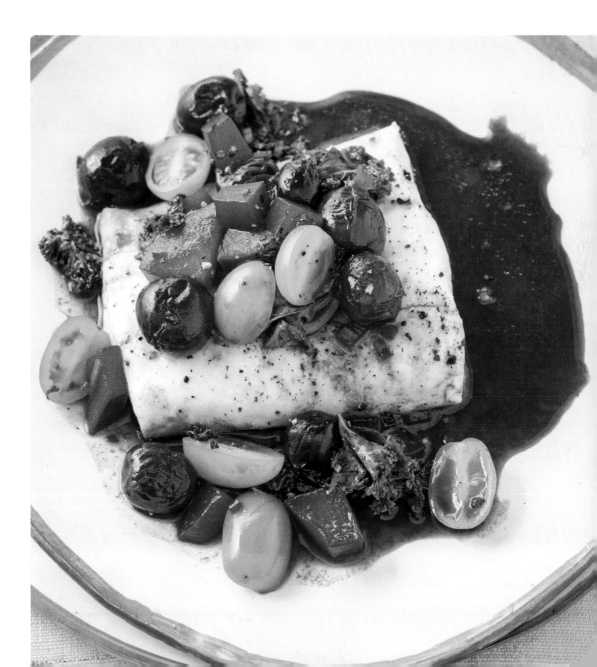

Butternut Squash Mac 'n' Cheese

I grew up on a steady diet of boxed macaroni and cheese (it was my dad's specialty: open box, boil water, and stir in mix). As I grew older, I still craved it, but the excessive dairy always made me ill. I've tried tons of vegan versions, and it wasn't until I played with butternut squash that I found success. This dish is ridiculous. My girlfriends are constantly asking me to whip it up. It's the ultimate comfort food without the payday that follows. Dig in!

1 butternut squash, peeled, cleaned, and cubed

2 tablespoons extra-virgin olive oil, plus more for drizzling

2 teaspoons smoked sea salt

2 teaspoons Cajun seasoning

16 ounces brown rice penne

2 to 3 shallots, chopped

2 to 3 garlic cloves, chopped

½ cup white wine

2 teaspoons mustard powder or Dijon mustard

1 cup unsweetened almond milk

1 teaspoon chipotle powder

3 tablespoons nutritional yeast

2 teaspoons paprika

2 teaspoons sea salt, plus more to taste

½ cup gluten-free bread crumbs

½ cup grated Parmesan (optional)

1 Preheat the oven to 425°F. Toss the butternut squash with 1 tablespoon of the olive oil, the smoked sea salt, and the Cajun seasoning. Roast for 30 to 40 minutes, or until soft. Leave the oven on.

2 Meanwhile, cook the pasta to al dente, following the package directions. Drain and set aside.

3 Sauté the shallots in 1 tablespoon of the olive oil for 3 minutes. Add garlic and cook for another minute. Deglaze the pan with white wine, cooking for 2 minutes and stirring

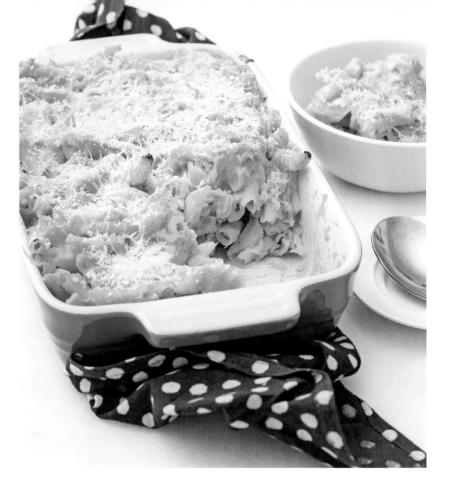

to scrape any browned bits into the sauce; stir in the mustard powder.

4 Combine the roasted squash, almond milk, shallot mixture, chipotle powder, nutritional yeast, paprika, and 2 teaspoons salt in a high-speed blender. Puree until smooth.

5 Grease a 4-quart casserole pan with olive oil or coconut oil spray. Add the cooked pasta and pour the butternut squash mixture on top. Mix well. Top with the bread crumbs, Parmesan, if desired, a quick drizzle of olive oil, and a light shower of sea salt. Bake the casserole for 10 to 15 minutes, or until the top is light gold.

Lazy Night Pasta

Anchovies are one of the ingredients that always made me squirm growing up. I thought of them as some sort of punishment food until I took the time to cook with them, and wow—these little guys really know how to bring the flavor! I'm always whipping up new pasta sauces, and this one featuring anchovies is now on regular rotation. This is a last-minute pasta or even a "make a good impression" dish whether it be your fifth or five thousandth date night.

16 ounces brown rice spaghetti

3 tablespoons ghee

4 anchovies

4 garlic cloves, sliced

4 Roma tomatoes, diced

1 (14-ounce) jar diced San Marzano tomatoes

2 teaspoons sea salt

pinch of black pepper

2 tablespoons julienned basil

2 tablespoons finely chopped chives

1 tablespoon chopped flat-leaf parsley

shaved pecorino cheese

1 Cook the pasta to al dente, following the package directions. Drain and set aside.

2 Melt the ghee in large saucepan over medium heat. Add the anchovies and stir with a wooden spoon until they have completely melted, or about 2 minutes. Toss in the garlic and cook for 1 minute, then add all the tomatoes. Sprinkle with the salt, pepper, basil, chives, and parsley. Sauté for another 8 minutes.

3 Transfer the pasta to a large serving bowl and spoon the mixture over the noodles. Mix well, adjust the seasoning to taste, add a dusting of shaved pecorino, and serve.

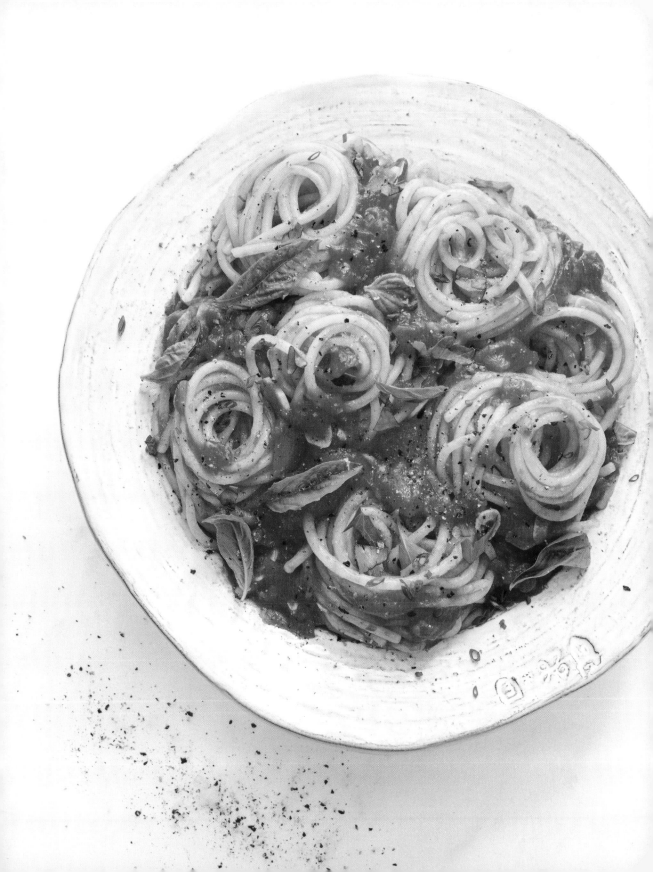

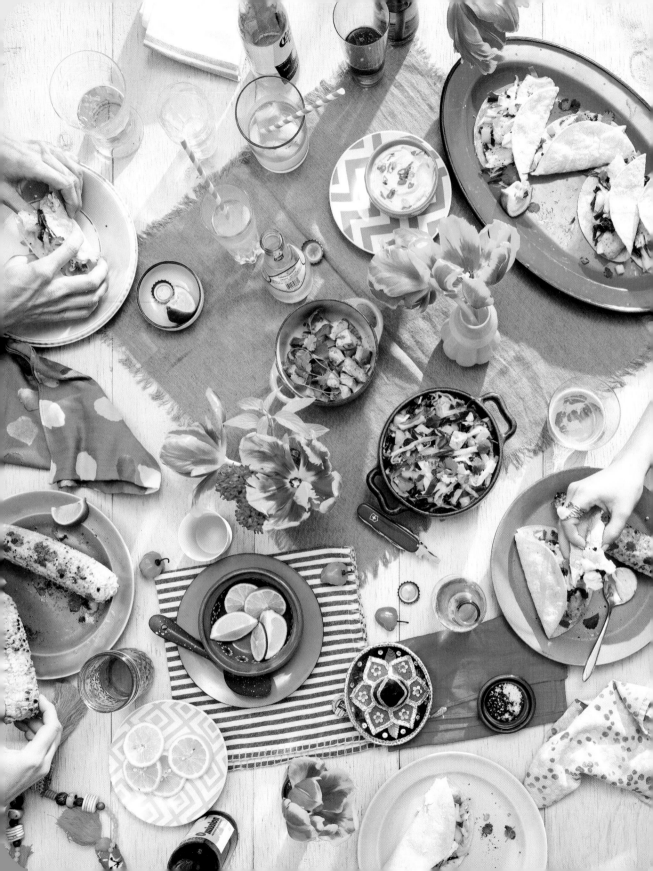

Fish Tacos

As a girl who lived in Southern California for eight years, I have had some seriously good fish tacos. Of course, the best fish taco I ever had was in Mexico, and that fateful taco inspired this recipe. You might want to sit down before you try the garlic sauce—it'll knock your sombrero right off. Don't be shy with adding the sauce—or even dunking your taco as you go! Enjoy this with some Korean Street Corn (page 183).

Garlic Sauce

½ cup soy-free vegan mayo
½ cup lactose-free sour cream
3 garlic cloves, minced
5 chives, chopped
3 scallions, green ends chopped
2 teaspoons sea salt
1 tablespoon spicy olive oil (such as guajillo oil, see Note)

Slaw

1 mango, diced
2 cups shredded cabbage (I use a purple and savoy mix)
3 green onions, thinly sliced
1 tablespoon extra-virgin olive oil
1 tablespoon soy-free vegan mayo
juice of 2 limes
1 teaspoon sea salt
1 avocado, diced

Fish Tacos

1 cup all-purpose flour or gluten-free flour
1 tablespoon spicy seasoned salt (I like Vulcan's Fire Salt from the Spice House)
3 to 4 (4-ounce) fillets of flounder, tilapia, or mahimahi (a good flaky, white fish)
2 tablespoons ghee
6 to 8 small gluten-free flour tortillas (I prefer Udi's brand)
spicy olive oil, such as guajillo oil, for drizzling
6 to 8 lime wedges for garnish
cilantro for garnish

1 To make the garlic sauce, combine all the ingredients in a blender and puree until the sauce is completely smooth. Set it aside.

2 To make the slaw, combine the mango, cabbage, and scallions. Combine the olive oil, mayo, lime juice, and salt and drizzle the mixture over the slaw. Mix well and then fold in the avocado.

3 To make the tacos, mix the flour and spicy salt in a large bowl. Dip the fillets into the powder mixture, one at a time, to coat them evenly. Melt the ghee in a large grill pan over medium-high heat. Cook the fish for 3 to 4 minutes per side, or until it is just cooked through and flaky.

4 Heat the tortillas in a lightly oiled skillet over medium heat, cooking them about 45 seconds on each side, until golden. Transfer the tortillas to plates and layer them with sauce, slaw, fish, a final dollop of sauce, and a drizzle of guajillo oil. Garnish each plate with a lime wedge and a few sprigs of cilantro.

Note: You can find dried guajillo peppers in the Mexican section of your supermarket. Place 2 roughly chopped dried peppers in 2 cups extra-virgin olive oil and heat the mixture over low heat for 20 minutes. Remove the peppers (but keep the seeds) and store in the cabinet.

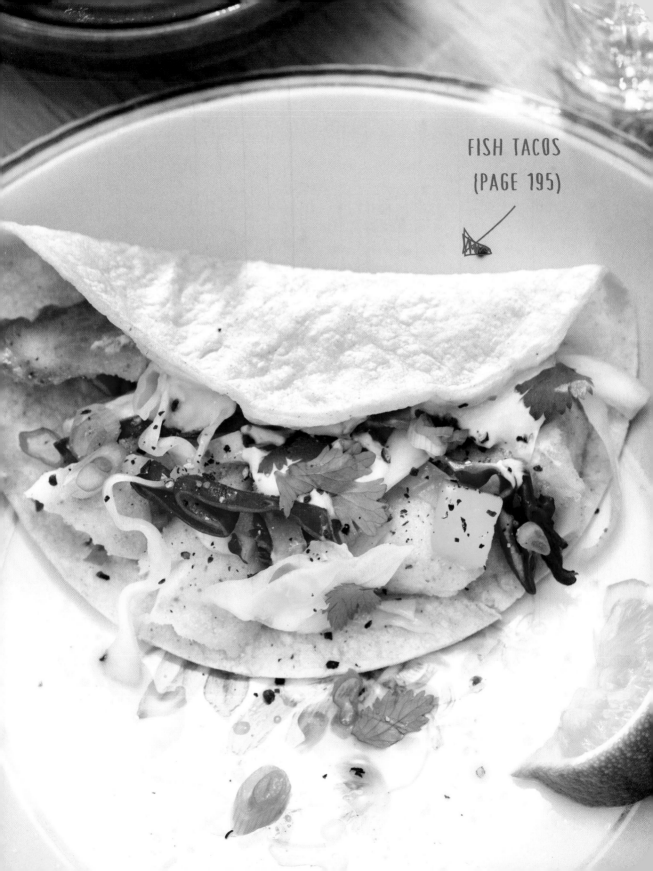

FISH TACOS
(PAGE 195)

Grilled Shrimp and Pineapple in Red Curry Sauce

MAKES 4 SERVINGS

You say curry, I say when and where. Curries are such a luxurious blend of flavors that have endless possibilities. You can alternate proteins (I often use salmon instead of shrimp for this dish), play with fire (drop in chile peppers till you cry), and let's not forget the mesmerizing fragrance of ginger, lime, and lemongrass.

2 tablespoons ghee
3 garlic cloves, minced
1 ½-inch piece lemongrass stalk, minced (see Note)
1 tablespoon paprika
1 teaspoon cumin
1-inch piece fresh ginger, peeled and minced
2 cups canned coconut milk
2 tablespoons red curry paste
2 bird's eye chile peppers (or red Thai peppers)
juice of 1 lime
2 tablespoons tamari
2 tablespoons fish sauce
1 cup dry white wine
1 pound small shrimp (about 20 shrimp)
salt

black pepper
1 cup chopped fresh pineapple
2 tablespoons raw honey or coconut sugar
3 sprigs fresh basil
rice or grilled bread for serving
cilantro sprigs for garnish
lime wedges for garnish

1 Melt 1 tablespoon of the ghee in a large pot over medium heat. Sauté the garlic, lemongrass, paprika, cumin, and ginger for 3 minutes. Pour in the coconut milk. Mix in the curry paste, chiles, lime juice, tamari, fish sauce, and wine. Cook over medium-low heat for 20 minutes.

2 Clean, devein, and remove the tails from the shrimp. (You can also have your fishmonger take care of this step ahead of time.) Heat the remaining 1 tablespoon of the ghee in a sauté pan over medium heat and cook the shrimp

until they curl and turn pink, 4 to 5 minutes. Sprinkle the shrimp with salt and pepper and add them to the curry pot. Stir in the pineapple, honey, and basil leaves.

3 Serve the curry over rice or with grilled bread. Top with fresh cilantro sprigs and lime wedges.

Note: If you can't find fresh lemongrass, you may be able to get a tube of lemongrass paste; this is often sold in the herbs section. Use 1 tablespoon for this curry.

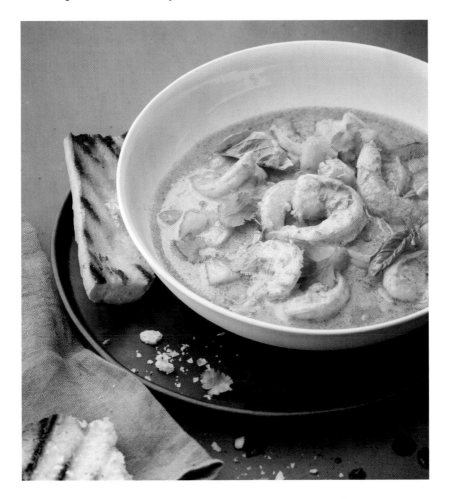

Orecchiette with Brussels Sprouts and Kale Pesto

I could eat kale and Brussels sprouts every day for the rest of my life and be a happy girl, but I know that not everyone shares my greens affinity. If you're trying to squeeze more green goodness into meals against the objections of your family or a stubborn partner, this is the perfect way.

Pesto

1 bunch curly kale, deribbed
½ serrano pepper (or other chile)
¼ cup pine nuts
5 garlic cloves, smashed
1½ cups extra-virgin olive oil, plus more if needed
1 teaspoon sea salt flakes
½ cup grated Romano cheese, plus extra for garnish

Pasta

16 ounces orecchiette
1 tablespoon ghee
2 cups Brussels sprouts, cleaned and slivered
1 teaspoon sea salt flakes

1 Bring a pot of water to a boil over high heat, then prepare a bowl of ice water and set it nearby. Toss the kale into the boiling water and cook for 1 minute; immediately transfer it to the ice bath. Drain the kale well and pat it dry.

2 Combine the kale, serrano, pine nuts, garlic, 1½ cups olive oil, and salt in a high-powered blender and puree until smooth. Add more oil if necessary to get the desired consistency. Stir in ½ cup of the Romano. Set the pesto aside.

3 Cook the orecchiette to al dente, according to the package directions. Drain and keep it covered.

4 Warm the ghee in a cast-iron skillet over medium-high heat, add the Brussels sprouts and salt flakes, and sauté for about 10 minutes, or until the sprouts are golden brown and slightly crunchy.

5 Toss the warm pasta with some pesto. (I use about ¾ cup for this amount of pasta, because I prefer a lighter dressing, but go according to what you love!) Gently fold in the Brussels sprouts, reserving a few for garnish. Serve with grated Romano cheese for sprinkling.

This recipe will make about 2 cups pesto, so you'll probably have leftovers. It will keep, refrigerated, for up to a week or can be frozen.

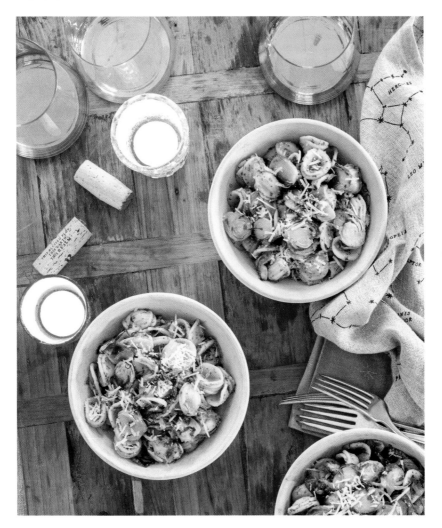

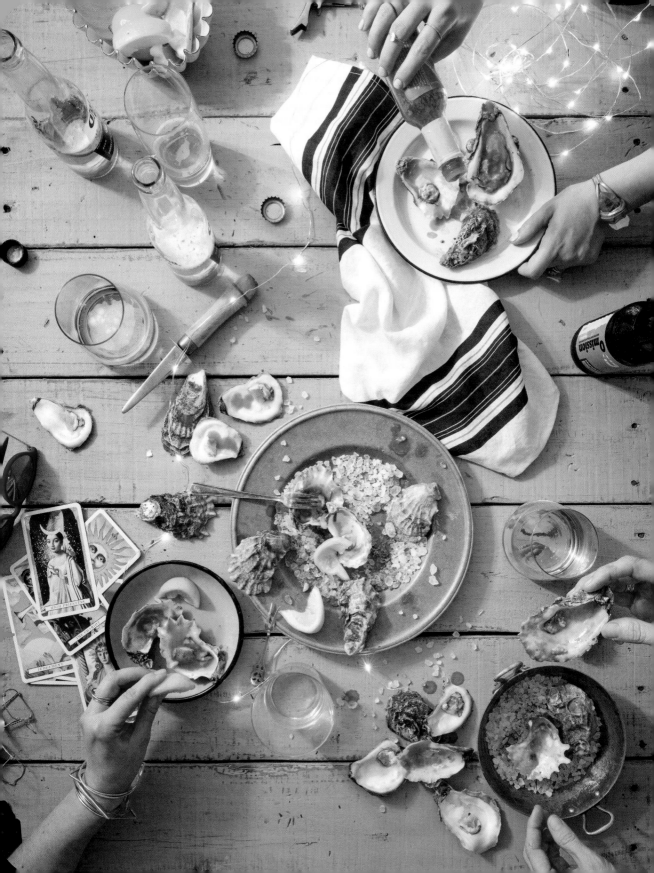

New Orleans-Style Charbroiled Oysters

MAKES 4 SERVINGS

They say it was a brave man who first ate an oyster, but a genius who threw them on the grill with butter and spices! I'm the first in line when you mention charbroiled oysters, and the best I ever had was of course in New Orleans. This is my valiant attempt to re-create the most delicious oysters I've ever had. Invite all your buddies over, because this dish is a party! And wear a bib—you'll end up slurping the sauce.

1 Melt the ghee in a large sauté pan over medium heat. Place the anchovy fillets in the ghee and gently mash until they become one with the butter, about 3 minutes. Transfer the mixture to a glass bowl. Whisk in the sriracha, hot sauce, garlic, red pepper flakes, sea salt, and lemon juice. Set the sauce aside.

2 Heat your grill or a grill pan to low. Shuck the oysters (see next page) making sure to clean the feet. Whisk the sauce well, place 2 teaspoons on top of each oyster, and place them on the grill for 8 minutes. Place another scoop of sauce onto each oyster and cook 2 minutes longer. Serve the oysters on a bed of coarse salt.

6 tablespoons ghee
4 anchovy fillets
2 tablespoons Spicy Sriracha (page 180)
3 tablespoons Louisiana Hot Sauce
6 garlic cloves, minced
½ teaspoon red pepper flakes
1 teaspoon sea salt
juice of 1 lemon
2 dozen fresh oysters
coarse salt, for serving

How to Shuck an Oyster

My husband is a wizard when it comes to shucking oysters, and he recently taught me how to crack these odd-looking shells.

What You'll Need

oysters
a hand towel
a shucking knife

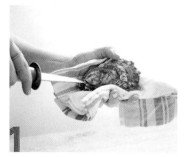

1 Clean the oysters under cold running water to remove all dirt.

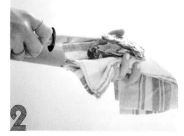

2 Tap the oyster before shucking (a hollow sound means they're dead and no good) and do a smell test (you'll know right away if they're bad). Discard any that are hollow, smell off, or are already open.

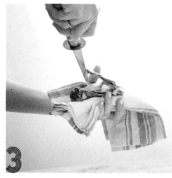

3 Hold the oyster in your nondominant hand in a hand towel, with the narrow part closest to you. Look for the "key hole"—that's the little notch where the two sides of the shell meet. Gently wiggle the tip of your knife into this notch until you hear it click.

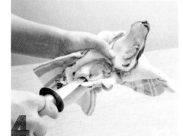

4 Assuming you are right-handed, turn your knife clockwise to pop the shell open. (Lefties should turn the knife counterclockwise.)

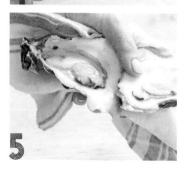

5 Slip your knife blade between the meat and the top shell to remove the feet. Do this on the bottom shell as well.

6 Voilà! Your oyster is ready to eat or to be popped on the grill!

Pollo à la Budig

My mother's specialty was chicken piccata. That lemony-salty goodness (as a kid I'd scrape off all the capers—little did I know I'd crave them as an adult) has become a Budig staple today. This sassy dish was born because I wanted to pay homage to the classic but give it a sophisticated upgrade. Thanks, Mom!

1 Preheat the oven to 425°F. Combine the flour and spicy salt in a large bowl. Dredge the chicken breasts lightly on both sides.

2 Melt the ghee over medium-high heat in a large skillet. Brown the chicken for roughly 5 minutes per side. Transfer it to a large (I use a 9-quart) Dutch oven.

3 In a clean skillet, heat the olive oil over medium-high heat and sauté the shallots, garlic, and serrano for 5 minutes. Deglaze with the white wine for 1 minute, stirring to scrape any browned bits into the sauce.

4 Pour the skillet contents over the chicken and add the tomatoes (with their juices), the lemon slices and juice, potato slices, coriander, cinnamon, capers, and Parmesan rind. Mix well.

5 Bake the chicken uncovered for 30 minutes, or until it is cooked through.

6 Remove the Parmesan rind before serving. Garnish with the cilantro.

1 cup all-purpose gluten-free flour

1 tablespoon spicy salt or seasoned salt

1 pound boneless chicken breasts

3 tablespoons ghee

1 tablespoon extra-virgin olive oil

3 shallots, minced

2 garlic cloves, chopped

1 serrano pepper, sliced

1 cup white wine

1 (28-ounce) can San Marzano tomatoes

½ lemon, thinly sliced

juice of ½ lemon

1 potato, peeled and sliced ⅛ inch thick

1 teaspoon coriander

1 teaspoon cinnamon

3 tablespoons capers

1 Parmesan rind

cilantro sprigs for garnish

Citrus Salmon in Green Juice

. . . .

This recipe was inspired by one of my favorites from my dear friend Giada De Laurentiis. She taught me the importance of using citrus with seafood (and pretty much everything). I followed her lead and added a modern twist of a green juice base and a creamy yet punchy topping.

. . . .

Green Juice

6 celery stalks
1 bunch flat-leaf parsley
1 bunch mint
½ lemon, cut into small pieces
1 bunch scallions, green parts only
1 tablespoon maple syrup
1 tablespoon white wine vinegar

Citrus Salmon

1 orange
1 Meyer lemon
1 grapefruit
1 cup flat-leaf parsley, roughly chopped
2 shallots, minced
2 scallions, whites and green parts slivered
6 tablespoons extra-virgin olive oil
1 (3.5-ounce) bottle capers
sea salt
4 (8-ounce) fillets of wild salmon
black pepper

Punchy Sauce

4 to 5 garlic cloves
7 ounces 2% plain Greek yogurt
¼ cup fresh mint leaves, julienned
sea salt

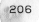

1 To make the green juice, run the celery, parsley, mint, lemon, and scallions through a juicer (a blender will work as well if you strain the mixture). Stir in the maple syrup and vinegar. Set the sauce aside.

2 To make the punchy sauce, mash the garlic in a mortar and pestle until it turns into a paste. Scrape it into a small bowl and stir in the yogurt, mint leaves, and sea salt to taste. Set it aside.

3 Zest the orange, the Meyer lemon, and half of the grapefruit and place the zests in a large bowl. Juice half of the orange and pour it into the bowl. Remove the pith and chop the remaining half orange, the whole grapefruit, and the whole Meyer lemon; add the chopped citrus to the bowl. Add the parsley, shallots, scallions, and 4 tablespoons of the olive oil.

4 Drain the capers and pat them dry with a paper towel. In a frying pan, heat 1 tablespoon of the olive oil over medium-high heat, add the capers and a sprinkle of sea salt, and fry for 3 to 4 minutes, or until the capers start to pop. Add the capers to the citrus blend and mix well.

5 Warm the remaining 1 tablespoon olive oil in a grill pan over medium-high heat. Season the salmon fillets with salt and pepper and place them facedown on the pan. Cook them for 4 to 5 minutes per side, depending on their thickness and how well done you like your fish.

6 To serve: Pour a small amount of the green juice into a shallow bowl. Lay the fish in the center of the pond and top it with the citrus herb blend, letting the sauce spill over into the juice. Top with a dollop of the punchy sauce.

CITRUS SALMON IN GREEN JUICE
(PAGE 206)

SHERRY MUSHROOM VEGGIE BURGERS
(PAGE 210)

Sherry Mushroom Veggie Burgers

I don't mean to brag, but these burgers absolutely rock! My husband is a huge fan of mushrooms served in a classic French sherry sauce, and I knew I could take the foundation of their deliciousness and turn them into an amazing veggie burger that any carnivore would adore. Make your life easier and cook the brown rice the night before (day-old rice works better) or pick some up from your local hot bar.

Lemon Vegan Mayo

1 cup soy-free vegan mayo

zest and juice of 1 lemon

2 teaspoons sea salt

Veggie Burgers

3 tablespoons ghee

2 teaspoons sea salt

5 shallots, diced

1 (15-ounce) can white beans, rinsed and drained

16 ounces mixed gourmet mushrooms (such as cremini, oyster, shiitake), chopped

1 tablespoon extra-virgin olive oil

½ cup sherry

¼ cup vegan cream cheese

1 teaspoon minced fresh sage

1 teaspoon minced fresh rosemary

1 teaspoon minced fresh thyme

1 cup cooked brown rice, at room temperature

1 egg, lightly beaten, at room temperature

¼ cup gluten-free bread crumbs

10 hamburger buns, halved

1 bunch mâche or watercress

1   To make the lemon mayo, combine all the ingredients in a small bowl and store it in the refrigerator until it's time to serve.

2   To make the burgers, heat 2 tablespoons of the ghee with 1 teaspoon of the sea salt in a large sauté pan over medium heat and sauté the shallots for 5 minutes. Stir often to prevent burning.

3   Add the white beans and sauté for another 3 to 4 minutes. Add the mixed mushrooms and olive oil. Season with the remaining 1 teaspoon salt. Cook for 5 minutes, or until the mushrooms are soft and have released their juices. Add the sherry and kick up the heat for 1 minute until it begins to evaporate. Stir in the cream cheese and herbs, and remove the pan from the heat.

4   Place the rice in a large bowl, then add the mushroom mixture and the egg. Stir in the bread crumbs. Let the mixture sit for 10 minutes, then shape it into 8 to 10 patties.

5   Heat the remaining 1 tablespoon ghee in a sauté pan over medium-high heat. Cook 3 to 4 patties at a time (being careful not to crowd the pan), for 4 to 5 minutes on each side.

6   Toast the buns facedown in the same pan for about 1 minute each, or until the cut surface is golden.

7   Serve the patties, topped with mâche, on the toasted buns spread with the lemon mayo.

Storing Herbs: While storing fresh herbs in reusable mesh bags works well, I prefer to do something that keeps them fresh *and* beauties up my refrigerator or counter. Find a beautiful mason jar and fill it with water. Place your herbs in the jar and either store it in your refrigerator or on your countertop. They're just as fragrant as flowers and uniquely beautiful.

Deconstructed Taco Bowl

When in doubt—taco night! Tacos are one of the best inventions known to mankind. I was going about my merry taco-making way one night when I realized I had forgotten shells. And voilà, this delicious bowl of deconstructed taco goodness was born. Who needs a shell, anyway?

Pico de Gallo

1 cup cherry tomatoes, chopped
¼ white onion, diced
1 jalapeño, diced
juice of 1 lime

Meat Filling

1 pound ground buffalo
Sea salt

Refried Beans

¼ cup chile-infused extra-virgin olive oil
2 (15-ounce) cans pinto beans, rinsed
1 tablespoon garlic powder
2 teaspoons sea salt
1 cup vegetable broth

Assemble

2 cups Coconut Rice (page 187) or cooked quinoa

2 cups shredded Bibb lettuce
Cashew Nacho Cheese (page 178)

1. To make the pico de gallo, combine the cherry tomatoes, onion, and jalapeño in a small bowl and mix well. Stir in the lime juice. Set the salsa aside.

2. Brown the meat in a sauté pan over medium heat for roughly 4 minutes. Season it with sea salt, then pour it into a bowl and set it aside.

3. To make the refried beans, using the same pan, warm the chile oil over medium heat and add the pinto beans. Season with garlic powder and sea salt. Fry the beans for about 5 minutes, stirring often. Slowly pour in the vegetable broth until the mixture becomes creamy, another 5 minutes.

4. To assemble the taco bowl, spoon some rice or quinoa into a large serving bowl. Follow with refried beans, buffalo, shredded lettuce, nacho cheese sauce, and finally, pico de gallo. Dig in!

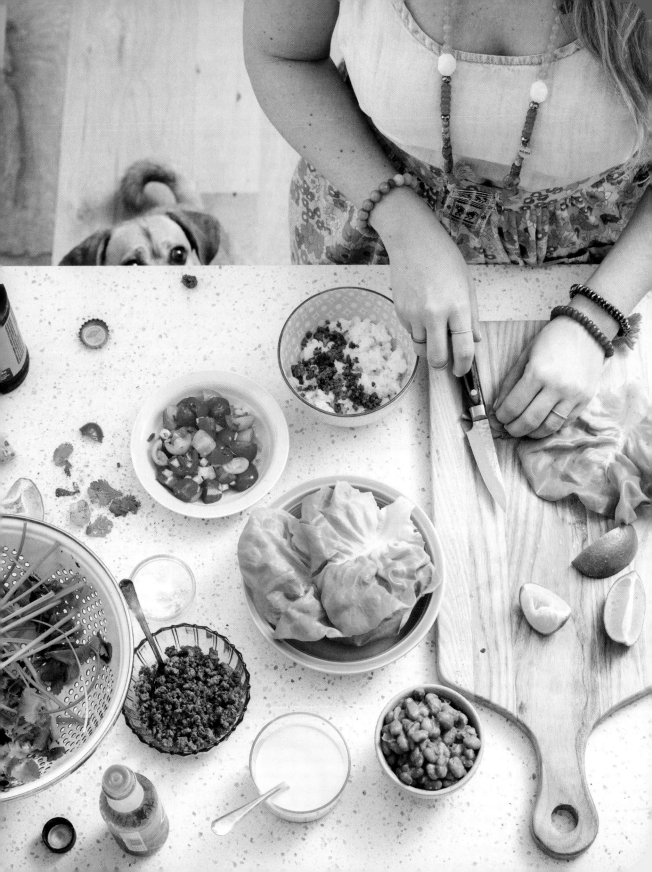

Mini Chocolate Chip Ice Cream Sandwiches

MAKES 6 SANDWICHES

I'm a total sucker for anything mini—and add ice cream and chocolate chip cookies to the equation? Sign me up! These mini love bombs will have kids and adults alike clapping their hands with joy.

Oatmeal Chip Cookies

½ cup butter

⅓ cup dark brown sugar

1 egg

1 teaspoon almond extract

1¼ cups almond meal or flour

½ teaspoon baking soda

1 teaspoon cinnamon

pinch of sea salt

¾ cup dark chocolate chips

¼ cup rolled oats

¼ cup unsweetened shredded coconut

Assembly

1 pint store-bought ice cream, or Maple Cashew Cornflake Ice Cream (page 223)

1 cup mini chocolate chips

1 Preheat the oven to 375°F. Place a silicone liner on one or two cookie sheets.

2 Beat the butter in a stand mixer or using a hand mixer until it is smooth. Add the sugar and mix for another 30 seconds. Add the egg and almond extract and mix until combined.

3 In a separate bowl, combine the almond meal, baking soda, cinnamon, and salt. Slowly add this dry mixture to the wet mixture on low speed until it is fully incorporated. Stir in the chocolate chips, oats, and shredded coconut.

4 Make balls of cookie dough roughly 1.5 inches in diameter and space them wide apart on a prepared cookie sheet, about two per row—there should be only about six on a sheet. (If you don't have two sheets, bake the cookies in batches, allowing the sheet to cool between batches.) Bake the cookies for 10 minutes, turning the cookie sheets and switching levels about halfway through the baking time: move the sheet on the top level to the bottom, and

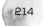

the bottom sheet to the top level. Transfer the cookies to cooling racks. Let them come to room temperature.

5 Place a scoop of ice cream onto a cooled cookie and press a second cookie on top to make a sandwich. Sprinkle the mini chocolate chips on the ice cream, dabbing them with your fingers to make them stick. Place these guys into the freezer for at least 20 minutes and serve them when you're ready!

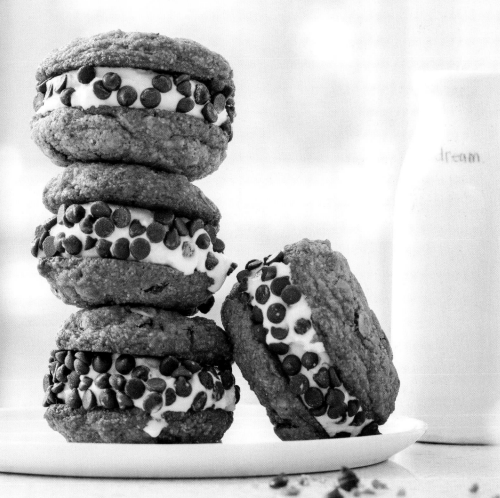

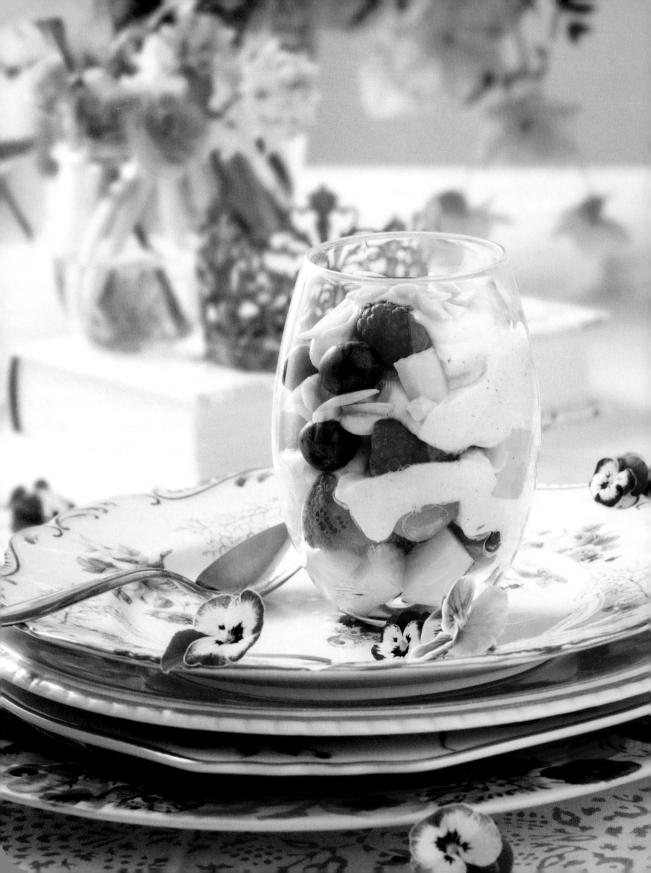

Fruitenstein with "Whip It Good" Dairy-Free Topping

MAKES 2 MONSTER DESSERTS

My mother used to make a version of this fruit salad for me when I was a kid, and I would happily devour it. It makes my mouth water to this day, but it was full of dairy and processed product like Cool Whip. So I got all mad scientist in my kitchen and came up with my beautiful, dairy-free creation—Fruitenstein! It's alive!

1 After you have finished whipping the vegan topping as instructed on page 181, but before removing it from the bowl, add the cream cheese, almond extract, strawberry yogurt, and lemon juice. Continue hand mixing until the mixture is well incorporated.

2 Layer one fruit group at a time into individual glasses, spreading a layer of dressing between each layer of fruit. Sprinkle a layer of slivered almonds about halfway through and as garnish on top.

Dressing
"Whip It Good" Dairy-Free Topping (page 181)
½ cup vegan cream cheese, softened
2 teaspoons almond extract
1 cup coconut strawberry yogurt (see Note, page 142)
juice of 1 lemon

Layering Assortment
¼ cup thinly sliced strawberries
¼ cup raspberries
¼ cup blueberries
¼ cup diced mango
¼ cup halved green grapes
¼ cup halved cherries
¼ cup slivered almonds

Peppermint Patties

My father used to keep peppermint patties in his refrigerator at his office. I would race to his stash every time I'd visit him, and to this day, the flavor brings back happy memories of hanging with my pops. This dairy-free version is not only a walk down memory lane—it's better than the original. It's a crowd-pleaser with kids and adults alike.

Filling

½ cup finely shredded unsweetened coconut

2 cups coconut oil

½ cup Powdered Sugar (see Sidebar)

½ teaspoon sea salt

1 tablespoon peppermint extract

Chocolate Coating

2 cups dark chocolate chips

solid part from 1 (13.5-ounce) can full-fat coconut milk

2 tablespoons dark rum or white crème de cacao

¼ cup coconut sugar

pinch of sea salt

1 Line a 9-inch loaf pan with parchment paper. Stir together all the filling ingredients and pour the mixture into the prepared pan. The layer of filling should be about ½ inch deep. Place the pan in the freezer for 1 hour.

2 Meanwhile, to make the coating, combine the chocolate chips with the coconut cream, rum, coconut sugar, and salt in a double boiler (or heatproof bowl set over, but not touching, a boiling pot of water). Stir often until the chocolate is fully melted and the mixture is smooth. Let it cool.

3 Using a 2-inch circular cookie cutter, cut as many disks out of the filling as you can. Let the remainder soften, reshape it into a ½-inch-thick layer, and return it to the freezer so you can make another round.

4 Line a cookie sheet with parchment and set a cooling rack on it. Using two forks, pick up a piece of the filling. Dip the filling into the

chocolate coating, then transfer the patty to the cooling rack and let it sit until the chocolate solidifies, 5 to 10 minutes. Repeat with the remaining filling.

5 Store the mint patties in the freezer and let them sit out for 5 to 10 minutes before eating.

Powdered Sugar: I find traditional confectioners' sugar to be painfully sweet, so I make my own version at home. Combine 1½ cups raw cane sugar and 2 tablespoons arrowroot powder in a blender and whiz together for 10 seconds. Store it in a tightly sealed jar.

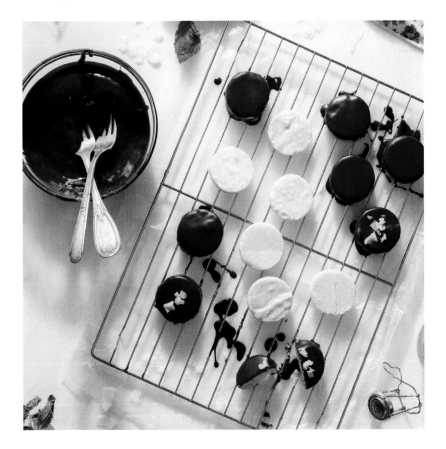

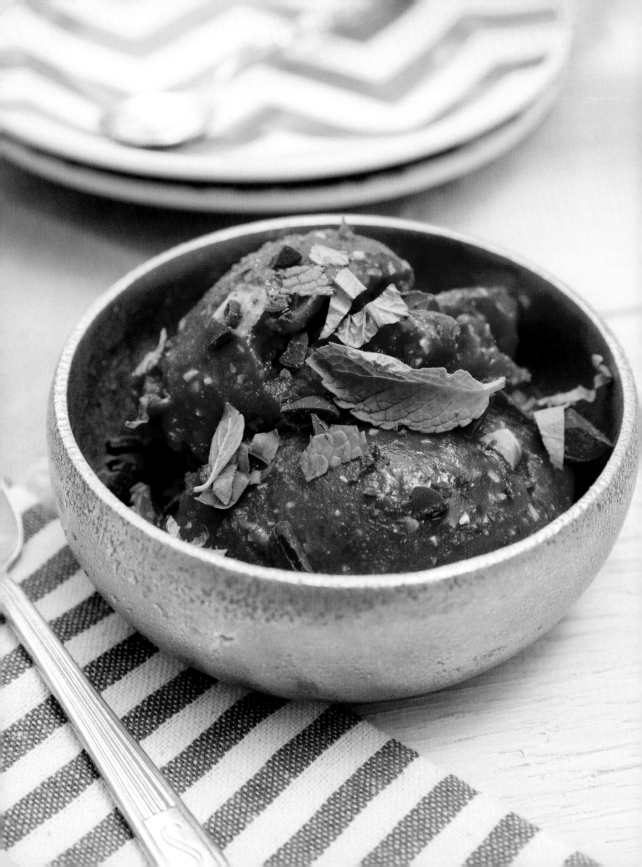

Cherry Coconut Sorbet with Chocolate and Fresh Herbs

MAKES 4 TO 6 SERVINGS

What's better than a guilt-free dessert? An easy and fast one. All you need are the ingredients and a blender, and you're ready to go! This is my favorite dessert when my sweet tooth kicks in or if I want to impress a guest on the fly.

1 Place the cherries and almond milk into a blender and puree until smooth. Add the coconut flakes and blend for another 10 seconds.

2 Scoop the sorbet into dessert bowls and top with basil, mint, and chocolate chips as desired.

1 (12-ounce) bag frozen sweet dark cherries
½ cup unsweetened almond milk
¼ cup unsweetened coconut flakes
chopped basil (optional)
chopped mint (optional)
dark chocolate chips (optional)

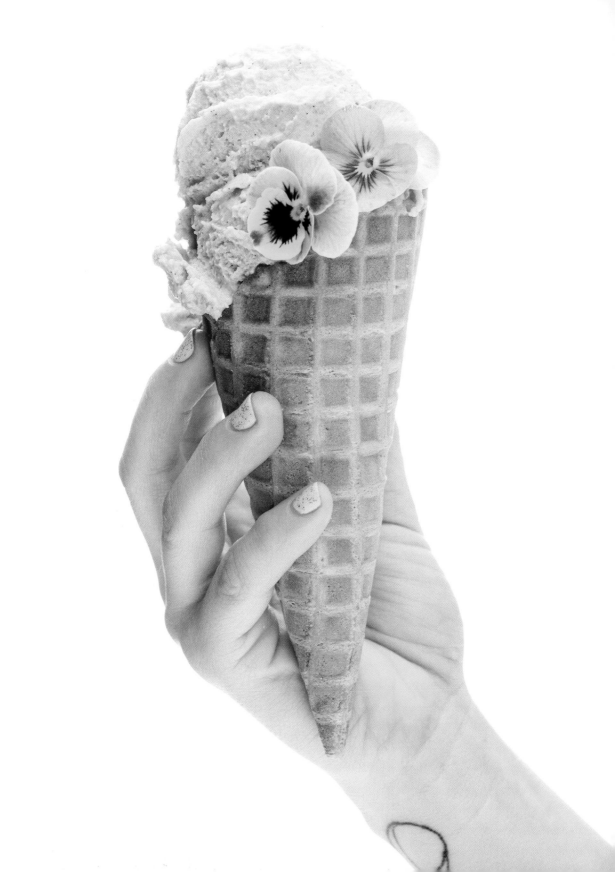

Maple Cashew Cornflake Ice Cream

MAKES 4 SERVINGS

I often daydream of an ice cream cone piled high with a swirl of soft serve—dairy-free ice cream is often lacking in the creamy department. While at a dinner party with dear friends in Belfast, I was served some amazing vegan ice cream. I snagged the container to see the main ingredient: cashews. Why hadn't I ever thought of that? I hit the kitchen to experiment as soon as I returned home and was not disappointed. Even my milk-loving husband went back for seconds. Okay, thirds.

1 Combine the cashews, water, coconut milk, maple syrup, maple extract, and salt in a high-speed blender and puree on high for a solid minute.

2 Strain the mixture through a nut-milk bag and return it to the blender.

3 Add the cornflakes and give a few pulses to incorporate them.

4 Pour the mixture into your ice cream maker and follow the manufacturer's instructions. Should be ready in 20 to 30 minutes.

1 cup raw cashews, soaked for a few hours or (better) overnight and drained

2 cups filtered water

1 (13.5-ounce) can full-fat coconut milk

½ cup maple syrup

2 teaspoons maple extract

pinch of sea salt

1 cup cornflakes

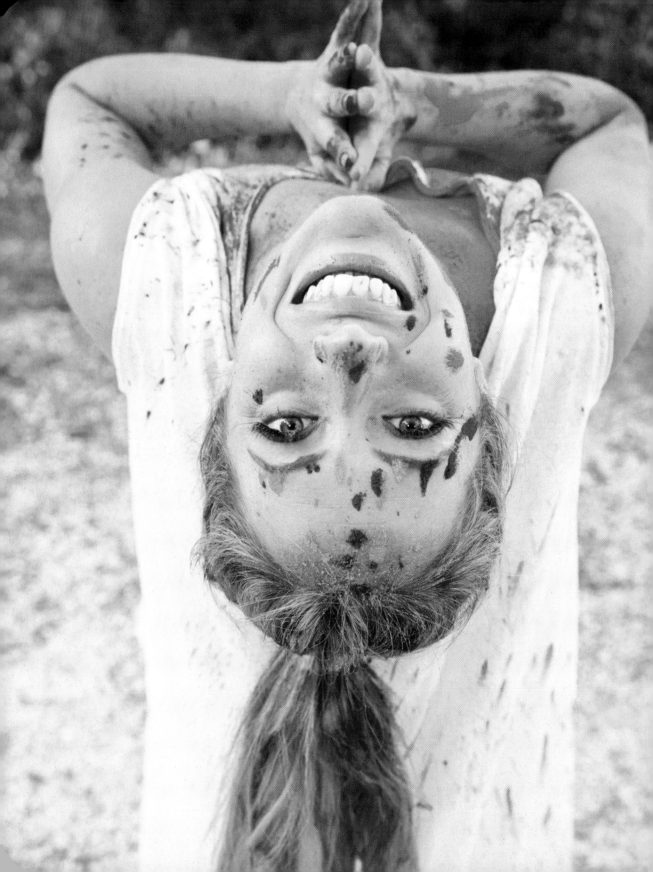

Nourish Your Spirit

I OFTEN SAY, BODY IS THE BOW,
ASANA THE ARROW, AND SOUL IS THE TARGET.

—B.K.S. Iyengar

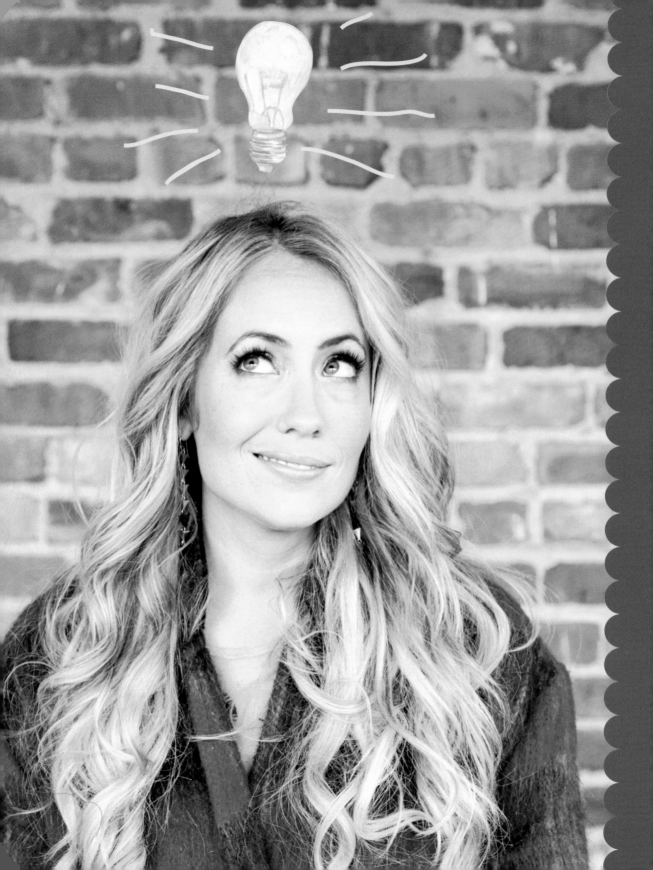

Eight

FLEX *the* MUSCLES *of* YOUR MIND

Consider this: You're like a big bowl of raw cookie dough. A big vat of multiple ingredients (agreements, talents, dreams, lessons) all lumped together in a confusing mess of dough. The flavor and potential is there. As you continue on your journey to aim true, you begin to take shape. This big vat of ingredients gets molded into individual balls (each representing a passion or idea). These balls of dough then get placed into the oven, where they must cook for the perfect amount of time—they can't be rushed! Time and the perfect heat (stoking your fire) is needed to form these balls into gorgeous, delectable cookies (that's right—*you*).

I started out as a little ball of cookie dough in Lawrence, Kansas, as a wild, imaginative Gemini baby. My father was the president of a university, and we lived on campus. I treated it as my vast kingdom. My mother would let me out of the house in the morning as long as I would make sure to be back in time for meals. All the extra space in between was filled with me and my imagination. This upbringing fertilized the seeds of my aiming true, even though I wasn't aware of it. I could be anyone I wanted in these times—Robin Hood, Maid Marian, Supergirl, a lawyer, an Olympic speed skater, an Academy Award-winning actress, and the list went on. I was a beautiful whirlwind of desires and dreams, unafraid to tackle any or all of them. I have my father to thank for this kind of belief system. I watched him go after huge careers that people would only dream of, and he always made them a reality. I watched him live this way and took note: if you want to do something—*do it.*

There's no task too big or small if it pertains to what you love. There's no room to fail, because every step along the way gets you closer than you were before. This belief system allowed me to stumble, succeed, and fall in many different arenas—I played every sport as if my heart would burst, I ran after a life onstage and on the silver screen, only to land on a yoga mat as a student with the natural gift of teaching. Do I think my purpose in life is to be a yoga teacher? It's a huge part of it, but in my mind it's only a piece of the pie. I continue to evolve in my personal and professional life, but know my underlying purpose behind every job or action that I take—it is my job to inspire, empower, and elevate those around me through my experiences, honesty, and ability to love. It may be at the front of a mat, behind a stove, or in the pages of a book, but I know my purpose, regardless of the chapter of my life.

Care to join me in this level of confidence? We've got to break through a few roadblocks before we dig deep into our purpose, so let's push any worry to the side and get to work.

What Have You Consented To?

If you want to find your purpose, you have to first understand your history and patterns. What beliefs do you have about yourself and your abilities? How do you define yourself? How do you let others define you?

People, opinions, and experiences can directly affect how we view our lives and what we consent to believe about ourselves. We possess the power to make change happen where we desire it. It's time to map out your patterns and self-beliefs (good and bad). Write down everything that you believe to be true about yourself—your abilities, talents, or lack thereof. It's time to look yourself in the face and acknowledge exactly what you're working with. Now write down as many qualities and/or stories you have consented to as possible. These answers will bring you closer to your purpose. Make a conscious effort to use your natural talents in your daily life and actions and to work on what challenges you.

What Treaties Do You Want to Break?

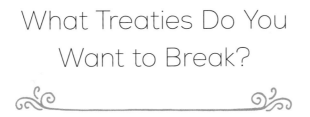

Years of experience create a vast web of storytelling that keeps us consenting to aspects of ourselves that aren't even based in reality. Time to break out of the prison that you've been holding the key to the entire time.

For example, I once auditioned for a yoga DVD, only to receive a personal phone call from the producer telling me exactly why I *didn't* get the job. She told me I was by far the best teacher for the job, but that she couldn't hire me because I had a tire around my waist. She said I needed to lose at least five pounds if I ever wanted to be camera ready, and continued to rip into me for the next forty-five minutes. This brief moment in my life became a demon who lived on my shoulder, constantly whispering little reminders about my unworthy belly and why I wasn't good enough. It took me years to beat this beast down, but by using *aim true* and surrounding myself with positivity, I broke back into a place of self-love.

In order to fully believe in ourselves and our abilities, we must destroy the beliefs that hold us back. Our purpose will drown in the sea of our fictional treaties, so let's throw out the life preserver and bring our purpose to life. False belief blinds us. Open up your eyes to see.

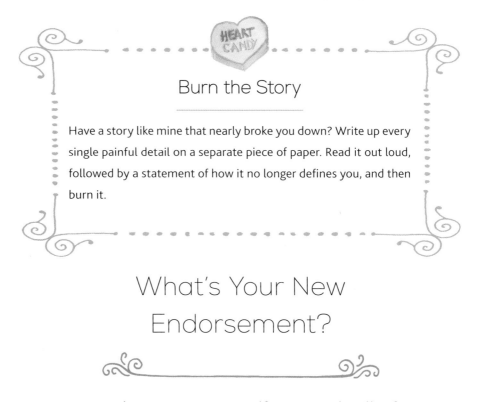

Burn the Story

Have a story like mine that nearly broke you down? Write up every single painful detail on a separate piece of paper. Read it out loud, followed by a statement of how it no longer defines you, and then burn it.

What's Your New Endorsement?

It's never too late to reinvent yourself. You are a bundle of unique talent, and you may get tangled from time to time, but you can always be rewoven into something magnificent.

Draw from the discoveries you made in chapter 1 to find your purpose and use what you have learned from the previous questions as a reminder: you always have the power to choose. Choose the life *you* want to live. Not the one expected of you. This may mean breaking a huge treaty that you've used as the foundation for your current life.

As terrifying as it is to demolish and start over, know that you need a foundation that is real, strong, and represents what you truly desire in this life. Surround yourself with support as you dive into the pool of change—envision success, know that road bumps are necessary and navigate them with finesse; be fearless in your choices. Set your aim, make it true, and stick to it with every ounce of your being.

Once you access the path to purpose, it's your job to keep the purpose fire burning strong by strengthening one of the most powerful tools you possess—your breath.

Just Breathe

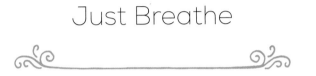

One of the most common phrases heard during stressful situations is "Just take a deep breath. It's going to be okay. Just breathe." Breath is a powerful tool when it comes to intense moments of stress or anxiety. It has the power to take us off the edge of the cliff and tuck us back into a relaxed state of mind. Breath is much more than a physical relaxation; it is the life force that keeps us alive.

Think of exhaling when it's cold out or of fogging up a glass with your breath. You know your breath is there—you feel it move through your body and give you life, and you can physically see it in the fog on your glass or your breath outdoors. It's way more than just moving CO_2 and oxygen—it's moving life force. The action of breathing is a subtle gateway to the world of our internal energy and life force. In practicing breathwork, we tap into our life force and influence how we want it to exist and be shared.

Our life force is challenged in stressful times, and we typically breathe too fast in these moments. Practicing deep breathing helps to trigger the parasympathetic nervous system, which brings us back into a state of calm and balance. This is the state we want to live in, but we can only do our best, considering life is full of surprises and often stressful situations.

So how do we slay the metaphorical lion and get back into a relaxed state of mind? Plain and simple: breathwork. The regular application of controlled breathwork will help soothe the overworked and stressed nervous system. The slowing of the breath will raise the carbon dioxide levels in your blood, bringing you back to a less alkaline state. This shift will help you trigger your parasympathetic state, thus lowering your heart rate and bringing you back to a place of calm.

Below I describe both heating and cooling techniques. Use the heating variations when you need actual heat in your body or a burst of energy. Use the cooling styles for when you need to calm your heart, body, and mind.

Heating Breathwork

VICTORIOUS BREATH (UJJAYI)

This style of breathing (which translates to "victorious") will be the most common if you venture into the yoga world. Ujjayi breathing is the simple action of breathing in and out through the nostrils with the mouth lightly closed. It is the style of breath used through the entire yoga practice unless a different style is specified.

How to:

* Find a comfortable seat and take a soft focus with your eyes.
* Start by breathing naturally with your mouth closed, perhaps even a slight parting of the lips.
* Deepen your breath by pulling on the inhale through your nostrils and then letting it swirl back out the nose on your exhale.
* Focus on a slight swirl in the back of your throat toward the top of your inhale, and a tiny extra push from the roof of your mouth as you exhale.

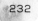 Aim True

Keep in mind: This is not nostril breathing. The nostrils are just the gateway for the breath to enter and exit. The actual movement is coming from the back of the throat, and the expansion of the breath fills the rib cage and not the belly.

You've probably taken a yoga class or two where someone's breath is so loud and dramatic that it pulls you out of your breathing and into their experience. My teacher always taught me that your breath should be loud enough for you to hear, but not necessarily so the person two mats from you can.

Where/when to practice: This is a calming and focused breath that helps you fall into the moment at hand. It's a simple way to shift your focus, whether you are at your desk or beginning your asana practice.

BREATH OF FIRE (KAPALABHATI)

This series of swift, forceful exhalations followed by a passive inhalation activates your diaphragm muscle like a mini punching bag, stimulating the core. The physical action of the abdomen is in and up. The tiny punching action forces the air out of the nostrils, like a panting dog.

How to:

- Make a fist and place the thumb side onto your diaphragm, or roughly around your sternum. Inhale deeply through the nose and softly exhale everything out.
- Inhale again and then begin a series of forceful exhalations, forcefully blowing out of the nose like an angry bull and using a swift, pumping action of the diaphragm. Exhale once per second.
- Focus your concentration on the exhale, allowing the inhale to come naturally and just quick enough to set you up for the next exhale.
- Practice three rounds of a minute each.

Keep in mind: The fist is there to help you with the action of drawing in and up in rapid movement.

When/where to practice: Kapalabhati can be done in many different poses when you want to build more heat (think Plank or Chair) or practiced traditionally in a comfortable seat. This breath is best used when you physically want to warm the body up, tone the abdomen (it's a surprisingly good core workout), or release pent-up energy or anger. The core is the home to insecurity, so stimulating it is a great way to bust through boundaries and move back to an empowered state.

Cooling Breathwork

4-COUNT BREATH

This is one of my favorite styles of breathwork and perhaps one of the most straightforward and accessible. I often teach this at the beginning of a class to help people focus or at the end of a class to help them relax and fully enjoy their Savasana.

How to:

- Find a comfortable seat or lie on your back. Exhale everything out.
- Inhale through your nostrils to a slow count of four. Hold your breath for another slow count of four. Gently exhale the air out your nose for another count of four.

Keep in mind: Start out the count in a regular manner, but as you become more familiar and comfortable with your breath, draw out the four-count. If you're looking for extra cooling, you can exhale through the mouth instead.

When/where to practice: Use this exercise when you need to slow down and be present. I've found this simple exercise to be one of the most convenient and useful breathing techniques to master.

ALTERNATE NOSTRIL BREATHING (NADI SHODHANA)

This style of breathing focuses on alternating inhales and exhales through the separate nostrils to create a full circle. The left side is considered the feminine or moon (*chandra*) side while the right side is masculine and like the sun (*surya*).

How to:

- Start seated and rest your left hand in your lap or on your left knee.
- Place your right thumb over your right nostril, fourth finger over the left nostril and index and middle fingers resting at the center of your forehead, or third eye. Your hand will resemble a tiny claw.

Close off your right nostril and inhale through your left. Once you reach the top of the inhale close off the left nostril and exhale fully through the right.

Inhale fully back through the right nostril. Close off the right and complete the circle by exhaling through the left nostril.

The goal is to always complete the four-part circle. It will look like this:

Left inhale . . . right exhale . . . right inhale . . . left exhale.

Or

Right inhale . . . left exhale . . . left inhale . . . right exhale.

When/where to practice: This is a fantastic way to balance out your thoughts and actions. If you know you need more cooling/feminine energy in your life (i.e., nurturing, open to receiving, calming), then start your inhales on your left side. If you need more fiery/masculine energy in your life (i.e., power, drive, confidence), start on your right side. Ideally this style of breathing will help you find the perfect mix to achieve balance in your life. It is easiest to practice in a comfortable seat.

TARGETED BREATHING

Here are a few simple breathing tips connected with everyday struggles such as anxiety and fatigue. Try these easy solutions whenever you need assistance!

Struggle with ...	Try This	Focus	How It Helps
ANXIETY	Lengthen your exhales.	Make the exhales symbolic of pushing out whatever holds you back, letting go of your shit, a literal sigh of relief.	The exhales trigger your parasympathetic nervous system allowing you to slow your heart rate.
FATIGUE	Lengthen your inhales.	Fill your lungs like a balloon. Envision that balloon light, buoyant, and free. Feel support and energy coming in with every breath.	Pulls in extra rejuvenating oxygen, energy, support, and heat.
ANGER	Practice Breath of Fire (page 233).	Sharp, fierce exhales cleanse the anger you've been bottling up. Let it all go!	Releases pent-up energy, allowing you to see clearly and make better choices.

 Aim True

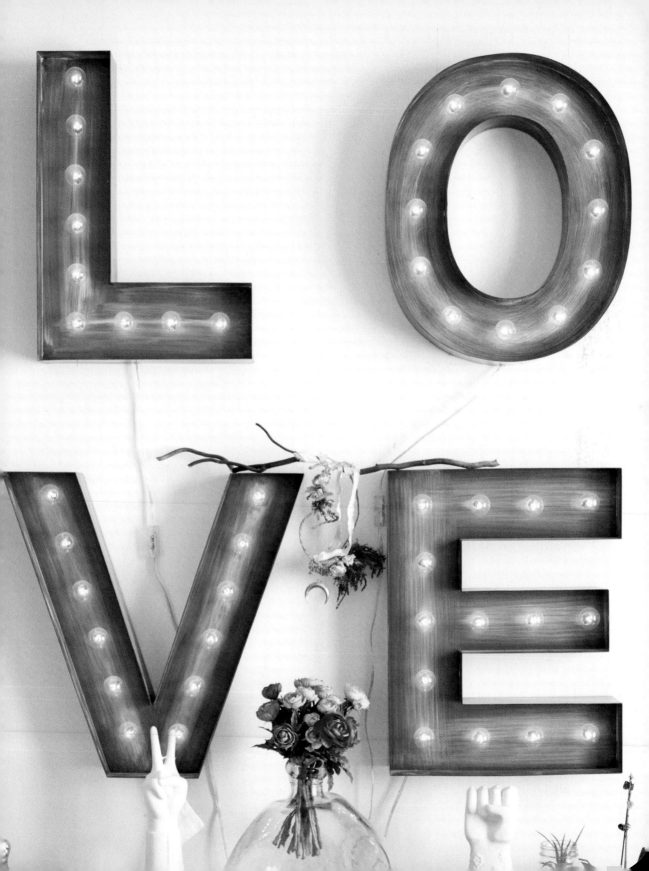

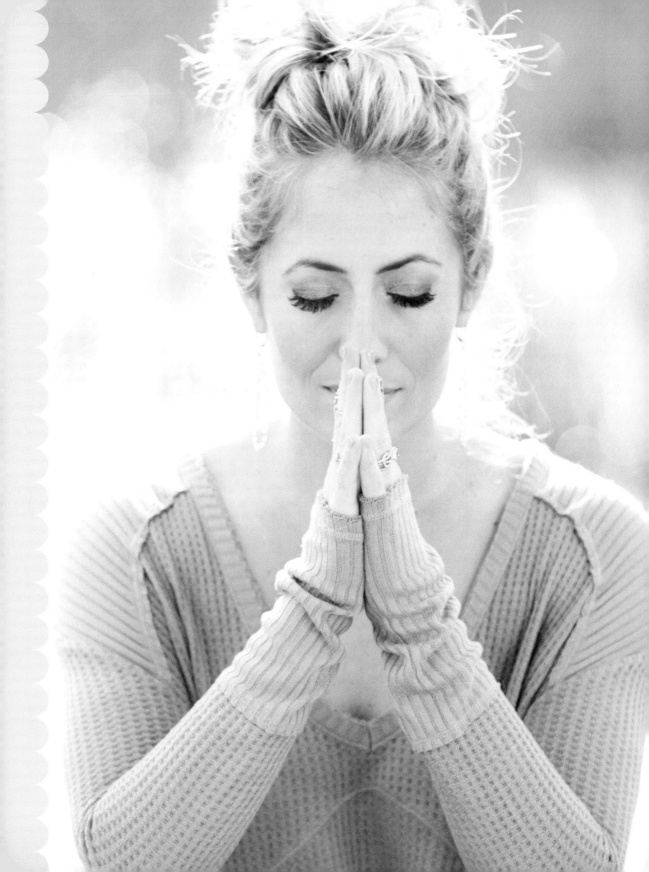

Nine

DEVELOP A MEDITATION PRACTICE

There's a common joke among those who meditate: if you say you don't have time to meditate, you should be meditating even more.

It is rather funny when we're too wrapped up in our own lives (and stress) to find five minutes a day to sit quietly (and feel way better). It's called excuses, and we are so full of them. The whole point of meditation is to study the self and how we act and react.

Step number one of finding a meditation practice is observing all the reasons why you don't have one:

I'm too tired.
I'm too busy.
I have no idea how to quiet my mind so why even bother?

I don't know about you, but that is just the short list of excuses I've used as crutches (and still use—I'm certainly not perfect, but a constant work in progress). Let's examine each item more closely:

I'm too tired.

Yeah, aren't we all? Life is busy, our brains are busy, and the result? We're totally worn down. But here's the thing. I'm not asking you to go sprint for five minutes; I'm asking you to find a comfortable seat and take five minutes to close your eyes, breathe, and slow down. This simple gesture can act as a lovely shot of caffeine to revive you and, hopefully, perk up your perspective so you can step back into your life revived.

I'm too busy.

I hear ya! I can't tell you how many days have blown by, and only when I curl under the sheets with my head on the pillow do I realize I didn't meditate. But was I too busy to not check my Instagram page? Busted. I guess I did have some time. The next time you sit down to do something mindless, remember you do have time to take a few moments for yourself and meditate.

I have no idea how to quiet my mind so why even bother?

Preach! Our minds are crazy, right? I'll try to sit and "not think" for a few seconds, and my thoughts are immediately like a bagful of Ping-Pong balls dropped all over the floor. The natural state of the mind is to think. Our goal through meditation is to slow down and clear the excess thoughts that get us into trouble.

MEDITATION IS JUST ONE INSULT AFTER ANOTHER.

—Chögyam Trungpa Rinpoche, Buddhist meditation master

Sitting with yourself and your thoughts can be harder than a class full of handstands and constant core work. Rinpoche's statement has always made me chuckle—meditation likes to talk major smack. I'm pretty sure he means meditation amplifies the way in which the ego shows up, which is major. For example, you'll tell yourself you want to sit for two minutes and clear your mind. It often goes a bit like this:

Sit tall. Breathe. Focus. Damn, I'm slouching. Okay—sit up! Hmm. I wonder what I'm going to have for dinner. Do I need anything from the market? No, no, no. Stop thinking. Clear the mind. Did I call Mother back? I know how much she freaks out if I wait too long. Dammit! FOCUS. Okay, okay. Breathing. What is that smell? God, I haven't vacuumed in a week. What a slob, this is so embarrassing. I can't believe I haven't—ARRRRGGG! Why is it so hard to stop thinking?!

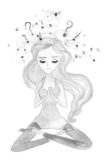

Welcome to your incredibly busy mind. It seems simple enough to sit and focus for a short while, and yet chaotic internal dialogues inevitably happen. When we sit and meditate, we awaken the beast, aka the internal state of mind. It's a window into how incredibly busy our thoughts are on a minute-by-minute basis and how pivotal meditation is to calm the circus.

Here's the problem: the ego is the master of ceremonies at the circus of your inner workings. It cracks the whip and makes the monkeys dance faster, because the ego doesn't want to believe in impermanence or that something as simple as focused sitting could challenge it. It rebels, creating chaos when all we want is a few golden moments of silence and connection. Luckily, we are now armed with yoga and breathwork to help quell the ego and its monstrous opinions, and to sharpen the body and our mastery of it. Dive into the breathwork as

 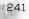

a natural tool to alleviate anxiety and calm the mind. All these steps help us find a state where meditation is possible.

Still concerned because you don't know how to do it? I got you. Read on for the best way to set yourself up for success, with plenty of different styles of meditation so you can find one that's best suited for you.

I realize it may seem like a big request to ask you to meditate every day, but I have my reasons. We're aiming to be disciplined, and this means consistency. Promise yourself to meditate for at least a few minutes per day. Once you get into the habit, it will become second nature, and then your mind will reap the benefits.

6 Steps to **Creating** a Daily Meditation Practice

. . . .

STEP 1: Find a space that beckons you to sit. You can meditate anywhere—even at your work desk, but the more time you take to create a space dedicated to meditation, the easier it is to drop the story and chaos from your regular life. Place a special pillow or cushion in the corner of a room and call that your meditation space.

STEP 2: Create a ritual. Treat your meditation practice the same way you would brushing your teeth: it's something that you need to do. Pick a regular time and keep it sacred. Try it first thing in the morning when your mind is calm and clear from a good night of sleep and ready to open to meditation.

STEP 3: Don't be attached to duration. One minute of sitting can feel like twenty, especially if you set a timer. If you want to develop this habit, don't be attached to how long you sit! If you long for more structure, there are some great meditation time apps that will start and end your meditation with ease (see "A Few of My Favorite Things," page 311).

STEP 4: Set a meditation date with a friend. Find a friend to sit with and encourage each other, especially when one of you isn't feeling so inspired. If you can't meditate together, text each other a yogic emoji when you have finished. There are also groups online or even apps where you can join a community, even see how many people are currently meditating.

STEP 5: Take notes. After you're done sitting, take a moment to jot down your feelings in your journal—how you felt before you decided to meditate, what kind of mood you were in, what kind of emotions came up, etc. Recording your experience and being able to look back on it will help you build the habit and stay accountable.

STEP 6: Pick your seat. There are endless ways to meditate. I've included several different styles below to get you started. Please try them all! Find the style that fits your life and inspires you. Make sure you sit for at least 1 minute and, beyond that, as long as you need. Happy meditating!

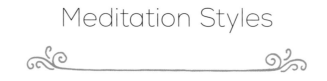

Meditation Styles

Mindfulness Meditation

This is the most basic way to meditate and can be one of the most challenging. There are no distractions, chants, mantras, or props—it's just you, your cushion, your breath, and your mind. (Oh, and your need to swallow. I'll explain in a minute.)

The goal here is to sit in silence and observe the mind. Does that mean you need to cease your thoughts? Not at all. Simply observe them and encourage the rowdy ones to simmer down and pass on through. The funny thing about this meditation is how, as you sit longer and longer, simple things become monumental. If you sit long enough, a pool of saliva will build in your mouth. For whatever reason, the action of swallowing it seems massive and disruptive, so you may find yourself holding the saliva and therefore obsessing over taking the time to swallow. When you finally do, it will seem so loud. Many small distractions like these will arise. Notice them, maybe even smile to yourself, then move on. Just keep sitting, breathing, and being in the moment.

How to:

- Find a comfortable seat (in a chair, on the ground propped up on a cushion, or even against the wall). Lengthen through your spine by rooting into your seat.
- Rest your hands on your knees palms up or down, or cup your palms in your lap with the palms facing up and the pads of the thumbs gently pressing into each other. Close your eyes and focus on your breath.
- Relax your eyes in their sockets and bring your internal gaze toward your third eye, or in between the brows. Focus on

easy, smooth breathing with the mouth closed. Notice the fluctuations of the mind but don't give them power. Notice them and let them pass.

* Continue to bring your energy back to your seat, your breath, and this moment, for as long as you like.

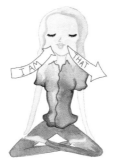

"I Am That" (Soham) Meditation

This is a simple and well-known meditation used in many traditions. It draws on the repetition of a mantra to help calm the body, quiet the mind, and align yourself with your intentions. *Soham* translates to: "I am that" (*so* = "I am" and *ham* = "that" or "the same as all"). "That" is determined by your personal interpretation, but generally refers to the object of one's meditation, whether that be a higher power or a quality. This meditation aids in dissolving perceived limitations and recognizing your true nature.

How to:

* Find a comfortable seat (in a chair, on the ground propped up on a cushion, or even against the wall). Lengthen through your spine by rooting into your seat.
* Rest your hands on your knees palms up or down, or cup your palms in your lap with the palms facing up and the pads of the thumbs gently pressing into each other. Close your eyes and focus on your breath.

Develop a Meditation Practice

- ❋ Breathe in and out through your nose with the mouth lightly closed. Make the breath full, but not forced.
- ❋ Once you've established a rhythm with your breath, start to attach your mantra. As you inhale, think *So* and as you exhale think *Ham*. Repeat this for as long as you like.

You can also choose to think in English if you prefer. Next, associate the meaning with each sound—every time you inhale, think *I am,* and every time you exhale, think, *that* (or *the same as all*). Start to connect your existence with every other being in the world. We all take these same breaths; we all experience the same emotions.

Continue to do this for 5 to 30 minutes. When you're ready to complete your meditation, join your palms together in front of your heart (Anjali mudra, page 38). Take a moment to absorb the meditation and any lesson it offered you.

INHALE	EXHALE
SO	HAM

or

INHALE	EXHALE
I AM	THAT

Find Your Mantra

A mantra is a word or sound repeated over and over to help bring concentration in our meditation practice. These mantras can be given to you by your teacher, picked up through a practice, or even created on your own. Here's a list of mantras to try out in your meditation practice. There are endless Sanskrit mantras, but some of the options in this list go beyond traditional Sanskrit.

Tat tvam asi. **You are that [which you seek].**

Om gam Ganapataye namaha. **Salutations to Ganesh, the breaker of obstacles.**

Om namah shivaya. **Salutations to that which I am capable of becoming.**

Om shanti om. **Om, peace, *om*.**

Om mani padme hum. **May I personally realize the jewel of consciousness that lies in the lotus of my heart.**

Kyrie eleison. **Lord, have mercy.**

Here, there, and everywhere. **The Beatles nailed this one.**

Aim true, stay true.

This is my personal mantra that I use when I do Japa meditation (see next page). It reminds me to not only embody everything in this book, but to stay dedicated to it through thick and thin. Think of words or statements that resonate with you personally or your current situation. For example, if you find yourself restless and frustrated, chant "I am grounded. I am calm." The options are limitless!

Japa Meditation

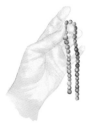

Japa meditation focuses on the power and repetition of mantras. These can be spoken aloud or spoken inwardly. Think of them as a repetitive prayer or intention setting. To assist with keeping count while chanting, the Hindu and Buddhist traditions use what Westerners think of as jewelry—mala beads. Malas have become quite trendy and fashionable in the yoga world, but they are traditionally used in meditation and prayer. A mala is made up of 108 beads (for 108 sun salutations, Upanishads, and marma points in the body) plus the "guru" main bead connected to the tassel, which symbolizes the lotus flower blossoming toward enlightenment. The beads are used for keeping count of the mantra in the same way that a rosary is when saying Hail Marys.

The beauty of this meditation is the power of sound, repetition, and charging an object with your intention. You can make your own mala beads or purchase some to help you practice using your mantra; the mala will energetically hold all your love, intention, and power.

How to:

* Take a comfortable seat (in a chair, on the ground propped up on a cushion, or even against the wall). Place the mala beads in your dominant hand, holding the first bead closest to the guru bead between your middle finger and thumb (the index finger is associated with ego, so we keep it separate from the meditation).
* Say/chant your mantra aloud or internally, focusing on the bead. Using your thumb, shift to the next bead, then repeat your mantra.
* Continue to do this until you have reached the final bead, the one that touches the guru (never meditate on the guru bead).

Targeted Mantras

Words are like the ingredients of a magical potion. When used properly, they manifest our wishes. Use these targeted mantras to help you overcome issues, feel empowered, and understand the importance and lesson of every moment.

Injury:

INHALE: I embrace this moment

EXHALE: Nothing is permanent

INHALE: I am open to receiving

EXHALE: I have everything I need

Trust:

INHALE: I'll see it

EXHALE: when I believe it

INHALE: I will stay open

EXHALE: to possibility

Connection:

INHALE: I have the power

EXHALE: I choose happiness

INHALE: I give love

EXHALE: I receive love

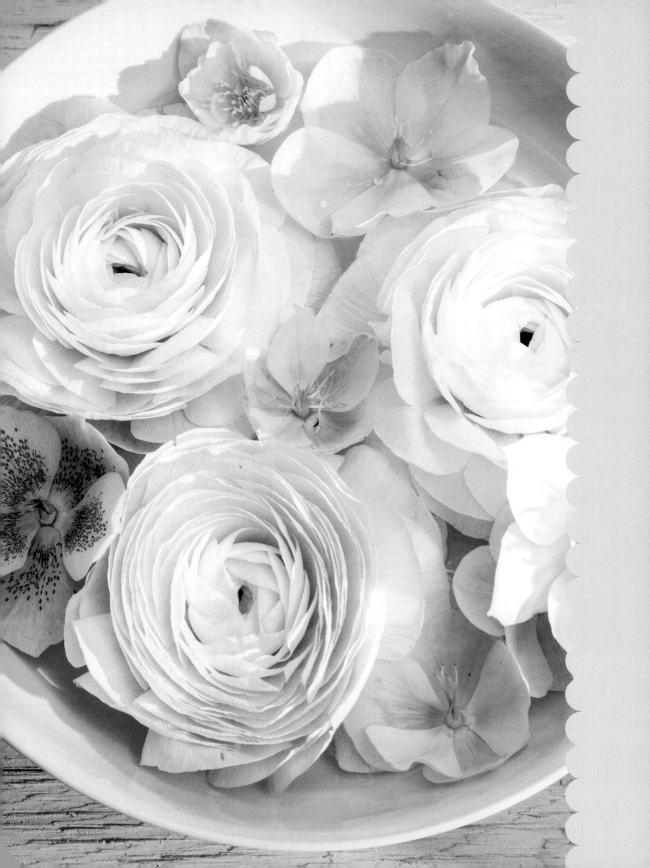

Ten

MOVE FORWARD
with LOVE

There are two simple choices in any given situation: choose to move forward with love or to retreat and react with fear. This lesson has been offered for years by many amazing leaders in the inspirational world, and it continues to hold strong. As cliché as it may sound, love *is* always the answer. Perhaps if we dive deeper into why, it won't seem like a generic platitude.

What are the most important components of your life? My heavy hitters are *relationships* (platonic, familial, and romantic), *work, food,* and *yoga*. These topics basically embody everything that's important to me. Now think about what's important to you and get ready to write your ideas down. I'll get the party started by sharing my topics and personal experiences. You'll see how easy it is to pick the fearful response, but that ultimately the loving response is your best option. Just remember that it's normal to hide in a place of fear, and that we're working slowly to climb out of that cave and in the direction that will reap you desirable results.

Always Choose the Loving Response

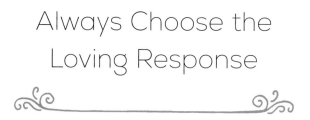

For now, write down your key topics. Underneath each one, create a column for Fearful Response and one for Loving Response.

Relationships

Write down three dramatic moments from the time line of your love life. Three heavy hitters in my life were:

1. Having a major fallout with my best friend of six years
2. Being lied to and cheated on by a boyfriend in a highly manipulative fashion
3. A relationship that ended without closure

FEARFUL RESPONSE

- Never trust again
- Close off emotionally from love
- Become jaded and bitter

LOVING RESPONSE

My first dramatic moment was like getting all the air knocked out of my chest. It's one thing to break up with someone, but another to lose a friend who's supposed to be there for you through thick and thin. While the heartbreak was palpable, the second this friend dropped out of my life, about four more doors opened. Once I shut the door on the relationship that was ultimately poisoning me, friends who now are like family walked into my life. My loving response was to wish her well on her way and recognize that I was exuding a light that wasn't similar to hers anymore. It wasn't a bad thing; it was just another step in our lives' evolution. Sometimes we evolve together, while other times, we grow apart and open the door to meet new like-minded friends.

Being lied to and cheated on left a deep scar. Everyone will have their heart broken at some point, but here's the beautiful news—it can't actually break. Go for a run, do a fiery yoga practice, bust out fifty jumping jacks—whatever will get your blood flowing! Do this, then take a moment to close your eyes and place your hands over your heart. Feel that under your hands? That wild little drum thumping away? That is your remarkably resilient and powerful heart full of purpose and determination. It beats and performs for you daily, no matter what. This feeling under your hands is your unbeatable will to aim true and love beyond any kind of limitation.

The relationship that ended without closure left me with questions and the time to learn that each of my poor relationships had set me up to fully embrace my husband once he came into my life. He wasn't the normal guy I'd go for, but that time I'd spent working through my experiences allowed me to see how perfect he truly was for me. Remember that each negative experience is just an opportunity to learn more about yourself and your needs.

My wish for everyone reading this book is to love fearlessly. Don't worry about the future—about whether you'll get married or have children. Take each moment as it comes. Fall in love with the person instead of the story you've written for them. If it works, fantastic! If it doesn't, mentally thank them for the lesson and move on. Everything you're given is a gift if you have the right eyes to see it.

Work

Write down three meaningful events in the history of your work life. Three experiences I have struggled with are:

1. Being up for a huge job only to have it taken away from me by someone else in the eleventh hour
2. Wondering if I'm good enough to maintain my job and make my students happy
3. Wanting to change my career path

FEARFUL RESPONSE

* Direct personal pain onto the person who got the job and try to tear them apart
* Doubt my abilities and constantly live in others' shadows
* Allow fear of rejection to take over and stay miserable in my current situation

LOVING RESPONSE

I think we can all relate to being up for a job that we know we'll be absolutely amazing for only to have it go to someone else, who clearly couldn't do it better—or perhaps we even find the person undeserving. The loving response here is plain and simple: there is enough work for everyone. If you don't get a certain job, all it means is it wasn't yours to start off with. Beyond that, it means that there is something better suited for you waiting around the corner.

Am I good enough? Do I have what it takes? These doubts are all too universal and apply way beyond teaching yoga. The truth is that there will always be someone who can do a job better than you, but here's the great catch—they can never do it like you. That's right. In the crazy huge world of ours, there is absolutely only one of you. Fabulous, quirky li'l you. Do you need to have Olympian ambitions or CEO talent? Not necessarily. You just need to own the talents you have and be unashamed of what they are. Your mind may always be peppered with doubt, but at the end of the day, you need to trust yourself. When you apply your skills at aiming true, you can rest assured that you're enough.

Maybe you want to change up your career path. Leave a high-paying job to be a yoga teacher, or pursue a dream you've had since you were a little kid. Fear can be all-enveloping here as you leave the comfort of your current situation in pursuit of the one you truly want. My loving response–life is an adventure! It's meant to be explored, challenged, and fully lived. Keep this mantra in mind as you step forward: I am adventurous. I am an explorer. I am up for the challenge. I will live fully.

Yoga

Write down the poses or elements of yoga that frighten you and–if you know–why. Here are three statements I hear regularly in the yoga room:

1. What if I hurt myself? I'm sitting this pose out.
2. I'm not flexible or strong enough.
3. Why is everyone else so freakin' good at this?

FEARFUL RESPONSE

* Avoid ever getting hurt by refusing to try anything new ever again
* Reinforce self-doubt by avoiding challenges
* Live in a constant state of self-doubt and competitive comparison with others

LOVING RESPONSE

When you're going for a pose you're unsure of, grab a small fort of pillows, place them at the front of your mat, and go for it! You've created a physical buffer to ensure you won't get hurt, and now it's time to tell your mind that a spill won't shatter your ego. We need the constant reminder that the only way to leave the nest is to fall a few times first. I'm not saying you have to tackle every pose that comes your way, but if there's a deep urge in you to understand it or learn the posture–keep on trying. Everyone deserves to feel the joy of strength, trust, and flight.

When it comes to doubting your strength, everyone in the world has thought or said this about themselves at some point. Remember, you practice yoga to gain strength and flexibility, not because you're already good at it. Don't let this worry you or drain your ego. It's a journey–don't be in a rush.

If you feel yourself about to ricochet into a long list of why the person next to you is stronger/bendier/more attractive, stop in your tracks and remind yourself of this: you don't know their story. They might have a wicked good handstand because it's the only thing they practice all day long, or they may have popped out of the womb hyper mobile. You just don't know. Choose the loving response by taking care of yourself instead of comparing yourself with those around you.

Stay True

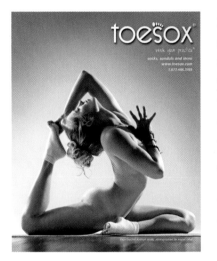

People constantly inflict their fears and insecurities onto others' dreams. (You want to leave your high-paying job to teach yoga?! Get a grip. You want to move to another country? Good luck getting the funds to do that! Do you even speak the language?)

If they can't understand it—or it threatens their view of themselves—they cast expectations. I had one life experience in particular that drove this lesson home.

I had been modeling for a company called ToeSox that ran their ads in the predominant yoga magazine every month. The ads got plenty of attention because I was wearing their socks. Just their socks. That's right—I was doing yoga in my birthday suit. The photographer for the campaign had shot an acclaimed series called *The Body as Temple,* which exhibited black-and-white nudes of dancers and yogis. His work was exquisite, and I was honored to be part of such a beautiful spread, celebrating the natural form and abilities that yoga and dance offer us.

The campaign was going swimmingly until a prominent teacher in the community wrote a letter to the editor, saying that she was disappointed in the magazine for their use of advertisement and nudity, and that she felt it was objectifying women. There was no mention of my name or ToeSox, but since she said advertisement, nudity, and *Yoga Journal* all in the same sentence, it was pretty clear that she was objecting to those very ads.

Next thing you know, everyone and their uncle came out of the woodwork to attack the ads . . . and me.

I'm so sick of seeing Budig's naked ass!
What a sellout!
These ads aren't yoga—they're just selling sex!

The comments went on, and I coiled deeper and deeper into my shell.

She needs to speak up! She needs to explain herself!

It took every ounce of self-control to not lash out at all of them, but I knew that wasn't the wisest move. So I sat on it. And meditated. I wrote a good old-fashioned pros and cons list of why I shot the campaign. Finally, I came up with my answer to everyone's statements: nothing.

I said absolutely nothing, and let me make this message loud and clear—you do not need to defend yourself to a bully. People will slam you with their fearful responses and opinions, especially when your actions don't line up with their beliefs. At the end of the day, the only thing you can hold on to is your belief, your ability to aim true, and your commitment to that intention no matter how many tomatoes get thrown at your head.

The expectations of others are meaningless. What truly matters is your ability to march forward with your beliefs and message regardless of how many people try to throw you off—and they will, oh, they'll try! Just know that people disagreeing with you doesn't make you wrong. It makes you unique and strong. Thank them kindly for their opinion and agree to disagree. If they can't handle that, then move on. Life is too short to focus your energy on those who don't support you. Look for your tribe (more on this in chapter 12) and the energy around you that is willing to support you no matter what.

Embrace Modern Spirit

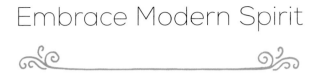

While the expectations of others will continue to swirl in the background of our lives and thoughts, a constant is our connection to spirit. If we can nourish the spirit by taking time for ourselves, we become stronger and better able to navigate challenging situations. Spirit can come packed with plenty of preconceived connotations. We all come from different backgrounds, religions, and beliefs, but at the end of the day, we're spiritual beings having a human experience.

When I say spiritual, I'm not associating it with religion but rather the ability to connect with who you are at your core, what you're made of, and how you connect to the people, energies, and environments around you. Beyond that, embracing modern spirit means carving out space for yourself to recharge, connect with yourself without the distraction of others, and manifest true balance. One of the best ways to cultivate a spiritual practice and take time for yourself is to observe ritual. Ritual can translate to anything sacred to you—stepping onto your yoga mat, taking the time to meditate every day, or even eating your favorite dessert in silence, reveling in every bite. You may not realize it, but all the Heart Candy sections in this book are tiny pieces of ritual to pull you back into a balanced and loving state of mind. Another fantastic way to chart your adventures into the world of spirit and self-care is through observing the cycles of the moon.

The moon is one of the most constant things out there—we know the moon will be in the sky every night, even if we can't see it. It follows a guaranteed pattern that serves as a natural calendar. People have followed the moon cycles for generations, and used its pull and power as opportunities to align their intentions. I suggest you follow these ways: check in with your intentions on the new moon and let go of anything that's holding you back on the full moon. Full moon is when the moon is in its full glory, and new moon is when the moon is preparing to grow again.

Artemis is the goddess of the moon, so I found myself researching the cycles as her prayer (page 3) took a hold on me. I started to keep track of where the cycle was and how it affected my energy and mood. It provided a beautiful way to check in with myself daily—I'd note the cycle of the moon, but more important, that was a moment for me to truly check in with my emotional state. I loved the ritual aspect of it, because it held me accountable for myself and reminded me to take steps toward constantly loving and bettering myself.

I offered my experience in a group ritual during one of my teaching trainings. We had been focusing on building our intentions and bringing them to life, and it just so happened that we were together on new moon. I asked if any of my students were interested in doing a new moon ritual, and everyone's hand shot up. A few hours later, we met outside, shivering from a mixture of the excitement and the brisk evening air. A few of my students had even adorned themselves in Artemis-esque tunics made from bedsheets.

I started the ritual by standing in the middle of the circle, lighting my candle, and stating my intentions for the following moon cycle. One by one, my students entered the circle, lit their candle from the person who'd gone before them, and spoke, until we had all shared our raw intentions and were standing in a glowing globe of soft, warm light. We had all given a piece of our soul and taken a sliver of everyone's energy back with us. Tears of release were shed by many, and to this day, that is one of the most powerful bonding experiences I've had with my students. I often get little love notes from them on new moon, telling me they're going to light a candle and set intentions. It makes my heart smile every time.

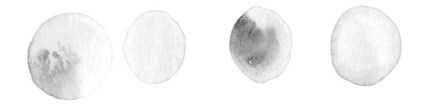

New Moon

The new moon is the opposite of the full moon. It's when the moon is seemingly gone—the sky is dark and the energy is heavy. The new moon marks the beginning of the waxing cycle building back up to full moon, a time of light and boundless energy. Imagine the new moon as an empty vessel. Envision what you want to fill it up with. It's a time of darkness, when you learn how to use your light.

GROUP RITUAL FOR A NEW MOON

Ideally this is performed outside at night, but a quiet place indoors will work too. Have everyone stand in a circle. One person begins in the middle lighting a candle and declaring an intention out loud. The next person comes in and lights a candle from the person who just shared an intention as that person returns to the circle. This continues until the circle is fully lit. The circle then blows out all the candles together.

When you express your intention, state what it is you want to move toward or into. What are you striving toward? What are you ready to let go of? What are your goals? The candles symbolize sharing your light and intention with your tribe. The inside of the lit circle represents the darkness and potential of the new moon, and the perimeter of light represents the full moon that will bring these intentions into action. Keep the candle after extinguishing it and take it with you to keep on an altar (page 47) or in a special place. Light it on the following full moon as a reminder of your vision.

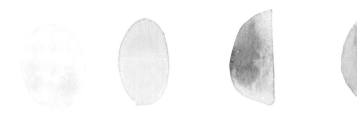

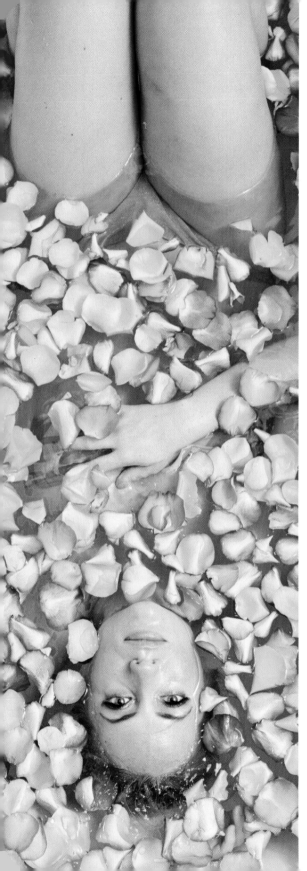

BATH RITUAL FOR A *New Moon*

Bath rituals are a fantastic personal way to find time to reflect, meditate, and get grounded. This soak recipe is my all-time favorite. I'll make it on new moon or anytime I need to feel grounded.

. . . .

10 drops vanilla extract or essential oil

10 drops orange oil

4 drops gardenia essential oil (optional)

½ cup powdered milk

1 to 2 cups Epsom salts

2 cups fresh herbs or flowers such as rose petals or lavender

Add the ingredients to a warm bath, one by one. Send your intentions into the mix so that they have time to marinate. You can also mix all the ingredients the night before.

Full Moon

Full moon is a great time to release something you need to get rid of or to celebrate an intention that has become reality. Moon energy is at its peak (think high tides, wolves howling), so get your tribe together and harness the moon's powerful energy. This is also an optimal time to do a forgiveness ritual because it's a time of releasing.

This ritual can be done privately or together as a group. Write down whoever or whatever it is that you need to forgive and place it in a fire-proof bowl or cooking pot. Burn the paper and say this over it:

I now release what I don't want, to make room for the desires of my heart. I now forgive and release everything and everyone of the past or present who needs forgiveness and release. I let you go!

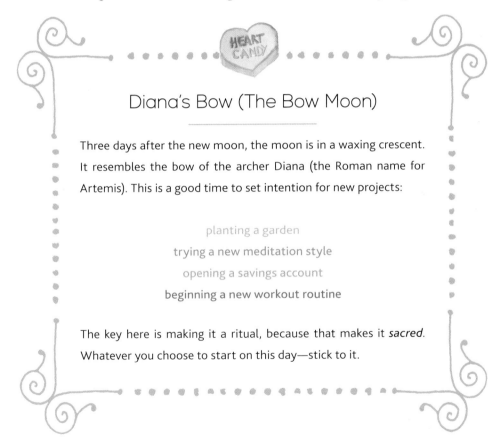

Diana's Bow (The Bow Moon)

Three days after the new moon, the moon is in a waxing crescent. It resembles the bow of the archer Diana (the Roman name for Artemis). This is a good time to set intention for new projects:

planting a garden

trying a new meditation style

opening a savings account

beginning a new workout routine

The key here is making it a ritual, because that makes it *sacred*. Whatever you choose to start on this day—stick to it.

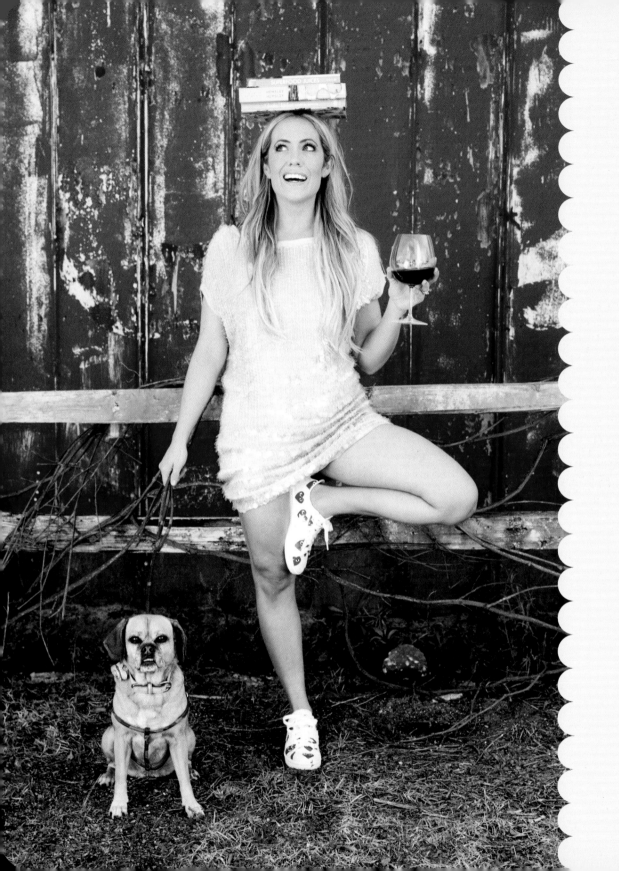

Discover True Balance

STEP WITH CARE AND GREAT TACT
AND REMEMBER THAT LIFE'S
A GREAT BALANCING ACT.

—Dr. Seuss, *Oh, the Places You'll Go*

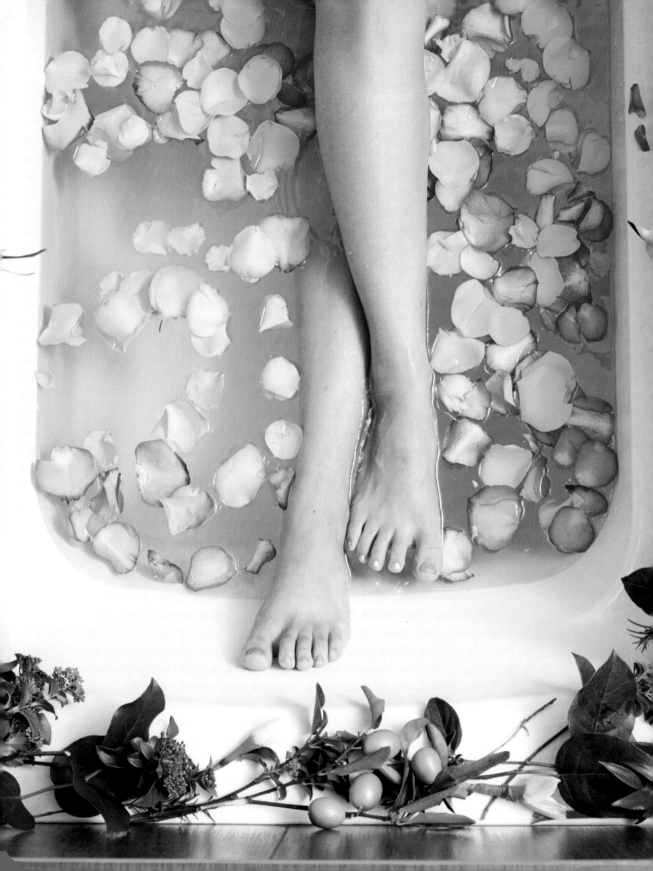

Eleven

Aim True at Home:
HOMEOPATHIC
SELF-CARE + BEAUTY
RECIPES

In a world full of deadlines, responsibilities, and expectations, one of the best ways to combat the chaos is to focus on self-care. Aiming true is all about finding balance—on your plate, on the mat, in your head, and now with your body. The body is a temple and should be treated with respect. It's a vessel that will weather with time, showing proof of lessons and adventures, but it's our job to keep it running in the best condition possible. What better way than to use natural and organic resources to help us along the way?

Let yourself be conscious and in charge of treating your body the way it deserves. The approaches below are meant to prevent and alleviate problems, while giving you easy and natural options for taking care of yourself.

Oil Pulling

Oil pulling involves swishing oil around in your mouth for twenty minutes and then simply spitting it out. This isn't about ingesting the oils, it's about using them to "pull" out bacteria that can cause tooth decay, gum disease, and other dental issues. I try to oil pull on a daily basis. While it's challenging to find scientific proof to back up these claims, about five thousand years (the practice is rooted in Ayurvedic tradition) and endless positive testimonies speak volumes.

Why you should try it:

whitens teeth naturally

promotes healthy gums

boosts the immune system

alleviates allergies

clears skin

decreases inflammation

What you'll need:

coconut or sesame oil

Give it a whirl:

1 Place 1 tablespoon of oil in your mouth.

2 "Pull" the oil by swishing it around your mouth for 10 to 20 minutes. (I normally oil pull while I'm getting ready in the morning and taking a shower.)

3 Spit the oil into the trash as opposed to a drain. (Otherwise it will clog your pipes over time!)

Dry Brushing

I'm constantly on the search for anything that will help me combat my allergies (sinus congestion, runny nose, and chronic sneezing). Dry brushing is one of the fastest ways to promote and kick-start a glorious flow of your lymphatic system. I always do this in the morning when I'm feeling drab and need to wake up. I recommend doing it one or two times a day.

Why you should try it:

stimulates the lymphatic system   reduces cellulite

exfoliates dead skin   perks you up

What you'll need:

a natural bristle body brush with a long enough handle that can reach those hard-to-get-to places

Give it a whirl:

1   Strip down to your birthday suit and begin brushing at your feet. Brush several times in each area before you progress up the body. Hit the lymphatic sweet spots like your inner thighs and armpits for extra lymphatic stimulation. Go gentle on your sensitive areas. Create long fluid strokes all moving toward your heart.

2   If you have time, take a warm shower afterward to stimulate blood circulation.

Activated Charcoal

This powerhouse toxin absorber has so many fantastic benefits, and when you use it for your teeth, it's also an instant way to freak someone out by smiling to reveal your black monster mouth! I always knew activated charcoal pills were a must-have on exotic trips in case you got sick, but I now brush with activated charcoal one or two times a week to maintain white, healthy teeth. I also appreciate its natural detoxifying benefits.

Why you should try it:

natural tooth whitener
powerful detoxifier

natural blackhead remover/
facial purifier

What you'll need:

a bottle of activated charcoal capsules (available at most
    natural food stores)
bentonite clay (for the face mask)
raw apple cider vinegar (for the face mask)

Give it a whirl:

1 **To try it as a natural tooth whitener,** remove the outer casing of one activated charcoal capsule and pour the powdered contents into a small bowl. Don't wear anything white! This can get messy, so lean over the sink and be prepared to wipe the sink down afterward. Wet your toothbrush and apply your normal toothpaste (I recommend natural brands without the added chemicals). Dab the toothpaste in the charcoal and brush as you normally would. (If you're hardcore, skip the toothpaste and just sprinkle enough charcoal on your wet brush to cover the top.) Don't forget to smile at least once at someone in your house while you're doing this!

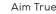

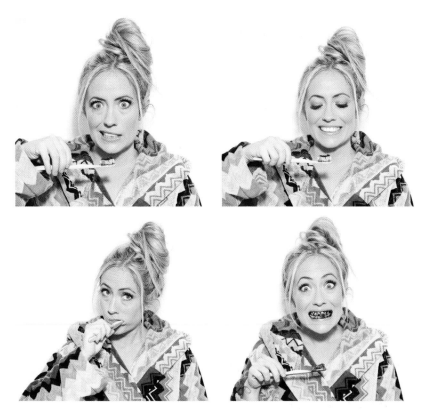

2 Brush as you would with toothpaste. Rinse out your mouth well (avoid swallowing the charcoal), and then brush again with a regular round of toothpaste.

3 **To try it as a face mask,** remove the outer casing of two activated charcoal capsules and pour the contents into a small bowl. Mix this with 1 teaspoon bentonite clay and 1½ teaspoons raw apple cider vinegar. Apply a thin even layer of the mixture to your cleaned face, avoiding your eyes and hair.

4 Allow the mask to dry for 5 to 10 minutes.

5 Remove it with warm water and a soft washcloth.

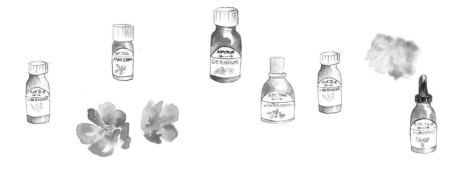

Essential Oils: The Cure-All

I can't remember a time before essential oils were a part of my self-care routine, nor do I care to. I have a vast collection of oils that bring me so much peace, joy, and comfort. I was originally turned on to essential oils by amazing body workers who would incorporate them into their routine. I began to associate the scents with feeling relaxed and rejuvenated, and once I realized their healing powers, I was reborn an oil believer. Here's a quick outline of my must-have oils and how to use them individually and together in blends that you'll never want to leave home without. There are tons of other amazing oils out there, as well as premixed blends, all with their own superhero properties. See "A Few of My Favorite Things" on page 311 for some suggestions, and read on for inspiration and to find what suits you best!

Note: If you have sensitive skin, you'll want to dilute the essential oils with a one-to-one ratio of essential oil to carrier oil (sesame, coconut, etc.).

Peppermint (anti-inflammatory, mood lifter, painkiller, sinus reliever)

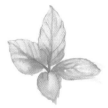

- Rub onto aching muscles for relief.
- Dab onto temples, hairline, and back of neck for headache relief.
- Inhale deeply or diffuse for allergy relief or an instant pick-me-up.

Wintergreen (anti-inflammatory, cooler, awareness enhancer, breath freshener)

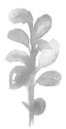

- Rub onto aching muscles for relief.
- Dab onto temples, hairline, and back of neck for headache relief (especially potent when combined with peppermint).
- Inhale deeply to lighten your mood.

Geranium (therapist in a bottle, antidepressant, refresher)

- Rub into soles of feet to calm agitation.
- Apply topically to relieve jet lag and physical stress.
- Inhale deeply to refresh your mind and spirits, and even alleviate PMS pain.

Lavender (cure-all, antihistamine, antibacterial, calmative)

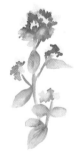

- Rub into the soles of your feet and neck at bedtime to help you unwind and ease you into peaceful sleep.
- Use as a lovely natural perfume or scent in deodorants and creams.
- Diffuse to provide a sense of well-being.

Marjoram (sedative, anxiety reliever, anti-inflammatory, antioxidant)

- Rub into the soles of your feet and spine at bedtime to alleviate insomnia or encourage restful sleep.
- Rub into sore muscles for pain relief.
- Diffuse to calm your mind and relieve stress.

Sleepy-Time Blend

This blend is part of my nightly ritual. The minute I smell it, my body knows to relax and sleep. Sesame oil has been used for years as a grounding oil, and the additional essential oils take it to the next level. It's a great oil to have on hand for restless nights or helping with jet lag.

¼ cup sesame oil
10 drops lavender essential oil
10 drops marjoram essential oil
5 drops Roman chamomile essential oil
5 drops orange essential oil
2 drops lemon essential oil
2 drops sandalwood essential oil
2 drops ylang-ylang essential oil

Combine all the ingredients in a dark glass bottle. Shake well and apply 1 to 2 teaspoons to the soles of your feet before bedtime.

Kick-the-Sick Blend

Using the proper oils is like calling in the troops when it's time to battle sickness. Each oil is a line of soldiers in my solid army of sickness butt-kicking. This mix is spicy and effective. Drop a bomb on your illness and bid it b'bye.

2 tablespoons sesame or fractionated coconut oil
10 drops oregano leaf oil

2 drops lemon essential oil
2 drops orange essential oil
2 drops clove essential oil
2 drops cinnamon essential oil
2 drops rosemary essential oil

Combine all the ingredients in a small bowl and mix well. Rub the mixture into the soles of your feet and let it absorb. Put on socks and go to bed or kick your feet up and let your little oil soldiers go to work! This can also be inhaled if you're traveling or around sickness. Dab it onto your neck and ears and put a pinch at the base of your nose when you want to keep sickness at bay. Store it in a small glass bottle or jar.

So Happy Blend

This blend is made up of some seriously happy smells—it's bright, vibrant, and alive. In fact, I just took a writing break to bust this blend out, and my fingers are now dancing on the board! Mix this up anytime you need to smile.

2 drops tangerine essential oil
2 drops geranium essential oil
2 drops Roman chamomile essential oil
2 drops ylang-ylang essential oil
1 drop ginger essential oil

Combine all the ingredients in a small glass bottle or jar. Drizzle five drops into the palms of your hands, rub your palms quickly, and take three deep inhales. Rub the oil into the back of your neck and onto your chest.

FINDING OM ON THE GO

It's often when we venture outside of our "typical" schedules that we need self-care the most. I have spent an ungodly amount of time on the road, and if there's one thing I've brought back with me (aside from colds and imported chocolate), it's how to travel like a champion.

Here's what to pack for staying calm and happy, even far from home.

Hydrate, hydrate, hydrate—oh, and moisturize:
- ✔ Eye drops
- ✔ Hand cream
- ✔ Lip balm
- ✔ Reusable water bottle

Pack the good snacks:
- ✔ Smoothie shaker cup with protein powder or powdered greens
- ✔ Homemade snacks such as my protein bars or granola (pages 146 and 149)
- ✔ Probiotics

Zen out:
- ✔ Ear plugs
- ✔ Neck pillow
- ✔ Travel outfit with layers and pockets

Create a home away from home:
- ✔ Small bag of Epsom salt to soak your feet and ease bloating
- ✔ Essential oils
- ✔ Travel humidifier
- ✔ Dry shampoo for staying glamorous on the road

Beauty Recipes

I love body and beauty products. Creams, toners, yummy perfumes, vibrant colors, soft shimmers, and everything in between. I was never one to turn down beauty products until it hit me: What exactly is in all this stuff? Have you ever read the label on a face cream? I had been conscious about what I was eating for years, and yet I wasn't paying the same attention to what I was putting on my skin—only the largest organ of the body. It was quite the terrifying epiphany. Let's not forget the cruelty aspect.

My nonprofit project, Poses for Paws, joined forces to support the Beagle Freedom Project, which woke me up to animal testing. I'm a huge animal lover and founded Poses for Paws as a way to help raise awareness and money for animals in need through yoga. We partnered with BFP, who taught us all about animal testing and how many companies test products on innocent animals, who are eventually destroyed after they can no longer be of use.

It opened my eyes further to the products on my shelves, and made me think about what kind of companies I wanted to support. This combination of cruelty-free and organic products got me thinking—what if I went all mad scientist in my own kitchen and whipped up amazing products that were tested on no one other than myself and willing friends?

Bingo. *Aim true* had made its way beyond the edges of my yoga mat and into my beauty products and self-care routines. And you know what? I loved it. It gave me an amazing education about natural remedies, how to use beautiful organic products around me, and, hopefully, how to influence others to do the same.

Coffee Scrub

This is insanely simple and always gives me glowing skin. Be careful: if you're sensitive to caffeine, you might want to do this earlier in the day, as I do feel an energy kick from it!

What you'll need:
1 cup used coffee grounds

Give it a whirl:

1 Bring the coffee grounds into the shower.

2 Wet your skin and then polish your entire body, including your face, rubbing in a circular motion. Rinse well and follow with a refreshing soap.

Deodorant

Okay, I'm not going to sugarcoat this: going from brand-name antiperspirants to natural is a rough transition. The goal is to wear deodorant without sweat-blocking and potentially hormone-mimicking aluminum, but without antiperspirants, you're going to sweat. I've found that there is a transition period of about a month dealing with odor, but if you can get past that—you're gold. It's totally worth it. Sweating is good and natural, and your body will thank you.

What you'll need:

2 tablespoons witch hazel with aloe vera

2 tablespoons vodka

5 drops Roman chamomile essential oil

7 drops eucalyptus essential oil

10 drops lavender essential oil

5 drops grapefruit essential oil

Give it a whirl:

1 Pour all the ingredients into a small (1-ounce) glass spray bottle using a funnel. Shake well.

2 Spray two or three times onto clean armpits. There may be a slight tingling sensation (which I find refreshing). Carry this in your bag and refresh throughout the day as needed.

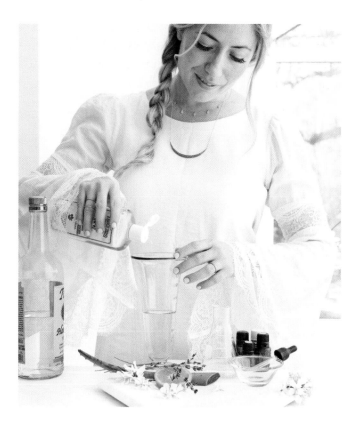

Brown Sugar and Lemon Body Scrub

This natural body scrub is as invigorating as it is delicious. Use it as a luxurious exfoliant; it will leave your skin feeling like butter and smelling just as edible!

What you'll need:

1 cup brown sugar
⅓ cup sweet almond oil
⅓ cup jojoba oil
7 drops lemon essential oil
15 drops bergamot essential oil

Give it a whirl:

1 Combine all the ingredients in a bowl and store the mixture in a mason jar for up to 3 months.

2 To use it, scoop a palmful into your hands and rub it in circles over your body. Continue until you have exfoliated as much as you want.

Face Serum

Serums give skin that dewy goodness, as well as nourishment that moisturizers don't always provide. Rosehip oil is the holy grail of facial oils and one of the only oils to contain natural retinol. Carrot seed oil has beautiful healing properties, while rose and jasmine are soothing, antiseptic, and anti-inflammatory, and improve the skin's elasticity. The rose and jasmine oils are pricier because they are so potent, but not to worry—a drop or two will go a long way, and a bottle should last you for a long time. As always, choose organic ingredients when possible!

What you'll need:

¼ cup jojoba or argan oil (or an even mix of both)

2 teaspoons extra-virgin olive oil

2 teaspoons rosehip oil

5 drops carrot seed oil

1 teaspoon vegetable glycerin

2 drops pure rose essential oil

2 drops pure jasmine essential oil

Give it a whirl:

1 Combine all the ingredients in a small cup and mix well.

2 Pour the mixture through a funnel into a small dropper bottle.

3 Before every use, shake the mixture well. Then squeeze roughly one dropperful into your palm and rub it over your face.

4 Apply in the morning and before bedtime.

Toner

I've always had sensitive skin, and I find if I wash my face daily, it tends to dry out, or even worse—break out. This toner is my answer to daily cleaning and toning. Geranium and lavender oil work wonders for the skin, while apple cider vinegar is a powerful cleanser and pH balancer. In combination, these offer antibacterial, antifungal, and antiviral properties. Great for daily use or clearing up problem areas.

What you'll need:

¼ cup raw, organic, unfiltered apple cider vinegar

¼ cup filtered water

20 drops lavender essential oil

20 drops geranium essential oil

Give it a whirl:

1 Combine all the ingredients in a dark glass jar.

2 Shake well before every use. Wet a cotton square and gently rub it all over your dry face.

3 Apply once or twice a day according to your skin's needs. Follow with a moisturizer or serum (see previous page). This keeps for up to 6 months.

Natural Blemish Buster

This simple blend can be applied to an oncoming blemish or one that's already reared its ugly head.

What you'll need:

2 teaspoons virgin coconut oil

2 drops tea tree essential oil

2 drops geranium essential oil

Give it a whirl:

1 Place the coconut oil into a small bowl and whisk in the essential oils.

2 Dab the mixture onto the areas that need assistance in the morning and before bedtime, but no more than twice a day. Store in a small jar for up to six months.

Sleepy-Time Pillow Spray

This recipe is so easy, and makes a perfect bedside companion. Spray it on your pillow nightly as a comforting ritual.

What you'll need:

½ cup filtered water

20 drops lavender essential oil

2 tablespoons vodka

Give it a whirl:

1 Combine all the ingredients in a mist bottle.

2 Shake, shake, shake before using! Mist it over your pillows before you go to bed to help you drift into la-la land.

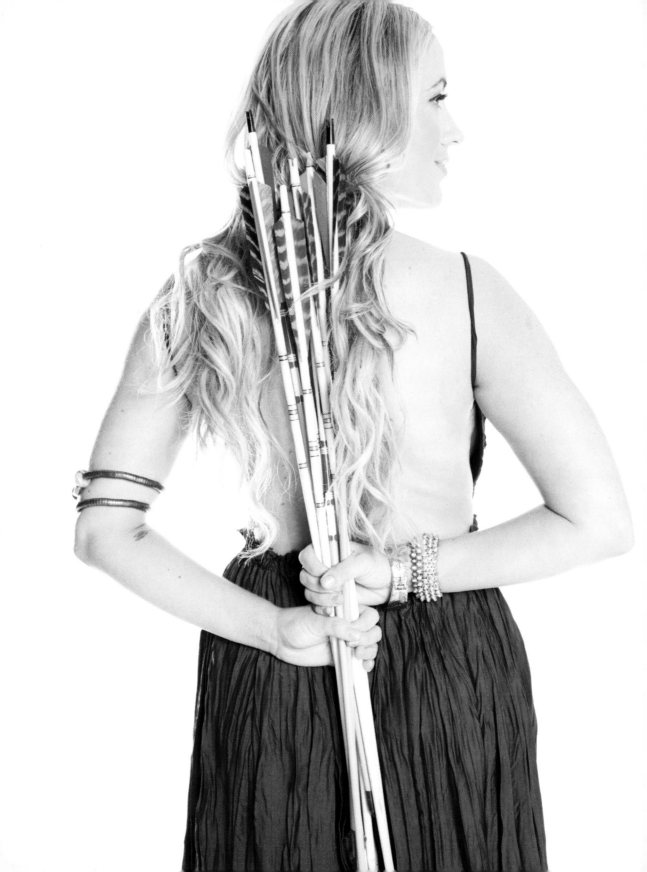

Twelve

NAVIGATE LIFE'S OBSTACLES

It's impossible to sign on to any form of social media these days without people tossing a dose of platitude potpourri out on how to navigate life's obstacles. The answer is not in a bulleted list or a slide show. In fact, the key to navigating life's obstacles doesn't actually have anything to do with the obstacles.

What we see as "good" or "bad" has more to do with what we bring to a situation and how we interpret it. Which is why the key to navigating life's obstacles is . . . to be yourself.

Being yourself means showing up equally on the days when you feel amazing and the days when you feel horrible. Be honest, give your emotions room to live, but don't tailor your personality to achieve approval or gain perfection. Magic happens in unlikely places and doesn't require a fancy top hat equipped with a white rabbit–it requires belief and dedication. Be yourself as you are right here, right now–in all of your glorious imperfect perfection. Strive to do your best, not for perfection. Know that some days are magical, while others are seemingly out to get you; don't let that rock your boat. Keep adjusting your sails in the storm so you can move in the direction you please. This is how you pull through the bumps of life.

The extra bonus of living this way? How you love yourself sets the example for how others can love themselves. Your ability to adjust on a bad day or shine on a good one gives people the belief system that they can do the same. Shine bright, but don't be afraid to be open and honest about the moments that frustrate you. Expose your rawness. Be honest with yourself about when you feel great and bad.

The Great Balancing Act

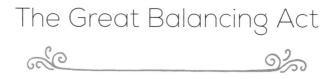

Have you ever been around someone who is so perky *all* the time that it comes across as insincere? Everyone loves a beam of sunlight, but a cloudy day from time to time is quite real, and even refreshing. The same variety applies to our attitudes—stay positive, aim to do your best, but allow yourself to have low moments. These moments are just as real and important as the ones we want to scream from the mountaintops.

I truly believe if more people behaved in this honest way, there would be less need to attempt perfection. We often see people's external shells that don't exemplify their internal motives at all. If we could just peel that made-up layer off and show that we're fabulous and flawed, everyone could breathe a deep sigh of relief and metaphorically take their bras off and unbutton the top button of their jeans.

We should seek out the same balance in our lives. Good days with bad. Success with failure. Ecstatic moments with periods of sadness. This may be easier to accept when you're on a winning streak, but as the king of emotion so aptly stated in Hamlet, "for there is nothing either good or bad, but thinking makes it so."

Nothing is good or bad—it's just the way we interpret our situation. That incredibly generous piece of the pie that allows us to shape our situations into a mind-set that is constantly favorable. If we can be

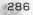

emotionally mature enough to not assume the worst in every situation, we're already a step closer to true balance.

So what is true balance? Being able to hold a handstand in the middle of the room without wavering? Rocking an amazing career that you love while holding down the fort with your family at home? Loving yourself and the people close to you? Eating a kale salad with a glass of red wine?

I believe that balance is all of the above . . . and more. Balance comes in many forms. We strive for balance in our physical body, balance in our discipline and work ethics, in our relationships, and even in our involvement with food.

True balance is knowing that it is always just that—a balancing act. I don't mean it's time to strap on your bejeweled unitard and walk the tightrope, but I do want you to have that level of commitment.

Balance means there's a chance you'll fall. The odds of crashing and burning are strong and, in a word, human. We all fall sometimes, but true balance belongs to the individuals who are willing to compose themselves and get back on the tightrope. Balance belongs to the yogi who is unafraid of the fall. You can't balance a handstand in the middle of the room until you've made peace with the possibility that you may fall out of it. The master of any craft has failed more times than the novice has even tried. This realization—that failure is necessary to gain knowledge and growth—frees us from the assumption that failure is terrifying or wrong. Obstacles are mere puzzles and those that leave us with a sense of failure actually give us the skeleton key to finding balance through success and failure in every genre of our life.

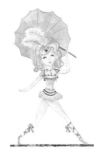

Balance Your . . .

What aspect of your life could use more balance? Check out this chart of challenges and discover ways to embrace the balancing act.

Balance	Challenge	Path	Tightrope	Embrace
Body	Your physical body will change every single day. There will be some days when you feel like a rock star, and others when you just feel like—well, a rock.	Push yourself to do better, but know where to stop before you push yourself over the edge.	Listen to your body, stay disciplined, and adjust your level of intensity accordingly.	Accept that today might be the perfect day to do a 90-minute intense yoga class or lift heavy weights, while tomorrow may demand a long walk with your dogs or even a day off from physical exercise.
Work/Life	Happiness doesn't lie just past the title of CEO or a certain number of accolades. There is no need for world domination.	Commit yourself to embracing your passion and helping to make a difference in the world.	Give yourself an attainable to-do list. Carve out the hours in the day that you're willing to dedicate to work, and decide what time to let the curtain fall on your checklist. Once you hit that limit, applaud your efforts and let it go.	One of the biggest differences you can make in the world is by loving the people around you. Set limitations for your daily workload to ensure that you get time in for the people and practices you love.

Balance	Challenge	Path	Tightrope	Embrace
Relation-ships	Love is a beautiful thing, but it can consume us if we're not careful.	True balance in a relationship never expects perfection, just honesty, commitment, and a constant reminder that you're always on the same team.	Learn to speak your truth and communicate even when you know it won't be easy. Speak from a loving and honest place and state your needs.	Communicate openly without fear, trust the other person implicitly, and know that there will always be highs and lows.

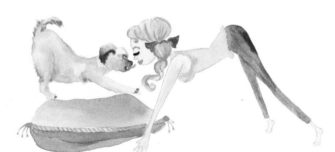

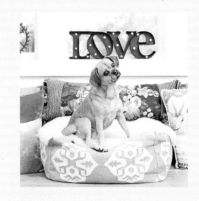
Find Your Tribe

So far we've analyzed individual ways to navigate obstacles, but beyond the self-work is the glorious opposite—finding your tribe. While I encourage you to do the work on yourself, know that you have and will work toward building a vast support system. You are never alone. Your tribe awaits you. I use this word because of its inherent ancestral energy. Historically, people form tribes as a way to create a unified family that gives them support and the tools needed for survival. This is how I view the friends in my life—as amazing tools for my soul's survival. A tribe is more than a group of friends; it is our roots.

A circle of energy that gives, nurtures, reflects, protects, and loves. A medicinal ground for celebration and truth.

Here's the catch—your tribe sisters and brothers will come and go. They all serve their purpose. They will enter your life right on cue, give you the tools and lessons you need to grow. You'll continue to evolve and grow together, or they'll complete their task and take a bow. The pain is just as real as the lesson, but what's most important is to understand that loving and leaving is a reality. With time, we find the people whose support and spiritual outlook will grow along with ours, but some will fall out along the process. This isn't failure—this is life. Aiming true will make your path clear and help you to see the friends who aren't as fully committed to themselves as you are.

It's physically impossible to find a human being who possesses all the qualities and attributes that you admire, need, and love. A tribe is a way of collecting all your desired elements into a group. For example, sometimes you'll need the friend who is constantly shining and optimistic when you're having moments of doubt. There's the friend who is brutally honest when you need a solid dose of reality and help getting your big girl/boy panties on. There's the quiet but good listener for when you need to vent and the comedian for when you want to laugh so hard you almost wet your pants.

Best friends have a little bit of everything, but your tribe will offer you the world. The friend who inspires you to jump out of a plane is just as special as the one who wants to cuddle all day eating cookies and watching marathons of your favorite show. A group of friends will offer you the support you need when you need it—someone to help pick you up when you're down, make you laugh over what once made you cry, or come bail you out of a bad situation, no matter the hour.

But—remember this—your tribe needs you as much as you need them. By offering your talents and true self, you summon others who not only need what you have to offer, but amplify your talents with the contribution of theirs. In a nutshell, finding your tribe and letting them find you makes the world a better place.

One of my best friends so aptly states, "You can never be the best version of yourself until you've found your tribe." It's like being a buried diamond who becomes polished by every member of the tribe. You become more brilliant, which only illuminates the beauty around you. We're all reflections of each other. When your aim is focused and true, you will pull in like-minded energy. It's crucial to do the self-work first, as anything less will attract confused energy, and often the people we don't truly want to associate with. Like attracts like, so open your heart to connection, kinship, and fearless support.

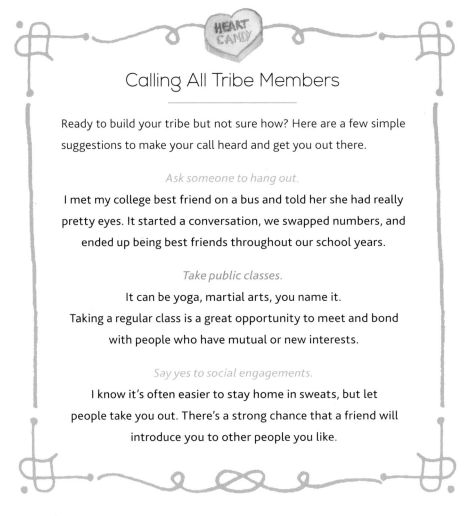

Calling All Tribe Members

Ready to build your tribe but not sure how? Here are a few simple suggestions to make your call heard and get you out there.

Ask someone to hang out.

I met my college best friend on a bus and told her she had really pretty eyes. It started a conversation, we swapped numbers, and ended up being best friends throughout our school years.

Take public classes.

It can be yoga, martial arts, you name it.
Taking a regular class is a great opportunity to meet and bond with people who have mutual or new interests.

Say yes to social engagements.

I know it's often easier to stay home in sweats, but let people take you out. There's a strong chance that a friend will introduce you to other people you like.

Likers Gonna Like

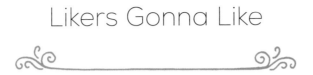

Fearless support is one of the most beautiful lessons I learned on my road to aiming true. My tribe taught me that support will always trump jealousy and competition. The single most powerful thing we can do as individuals is support the others around us—especially those we see as competition.

I learned this lesson at an early age from a remarkable woman named Seane Corn. Seane is a legend in the yoga world and rightly so—she is a living Wonder Woman who is selfless, fearless, and straight-up kick-ass. I adore her and consider her to be my yoga mentor/sister, but once upon a time, I knew her only from the pages of magazines. She started taking my morning classes (it's a miracle I didn't pass out from intimidation), and I eventually asked her out for lunch to see if I could pick her brain.

She agreed, with one condition—she was willing to teach me anything and everything I wanted to know, as long as I promised to do the same when someone asked it of me. Especially if that person threatened or intimidated me. I gave her a wide-eyed bob of my head, and the beginning of an amazing mentorship was born.

Seane could have viewed me as competition, but instead opened her world and heart to me. Seane taught me that collaboration and support is the only way to succeed, especially among a sea of sharks looking to devour one another to stay at the top of the food chain. Has either one of us ever threatened each other's career? Of course not. She rocks the world in her unique way and, through her mentorship, has generously offered me the keys to do the same.

Step Outside Your Comfort Zone

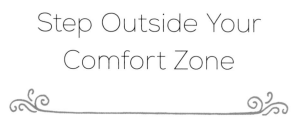

This chapter broke down how to navigate life's obstacles, but sometimes you actually need to summon them. Had I never grown the balls to ask Seane Corn out to lunch, I would have never absorbed valuable lessons that I use every day of my life. For Seane, had she chosen to see me as competition, she may have never taken my class in the first place! We need to learn to step outside of comfort zones in order to grow, and this often means facing obstacles with confidence and compassion. In the words of journalist Mary Schmich, "Do one thing every day that scares you." Here's a short list of ways to tackle daily fears and end up on top:

✔ *Be proactive.* Ask a love/friend interest out to lunch. You'll never know if you never try! It could be the beginning of quite the life/love affair.

✔ *Say what you need to say.* Speak up on subjects that matter to you, even if you fear rejection. Don't just sit on your golden egg to protect it—speak up and fight for it!

✔ *Do something outside of the box.* Take a trapeze class! The idea of swinging into the unknown might terrify you, but take the plunge. You'll realize there's a real and metaphorical net always waiting to catch you when you fall.

✔ *Take yourself on a date.* You don't need another person to give you permission to go out and have a good time! Take yourself on a picnic, cuddle up to your favorite restaurant at the bar, go lounge at the dog park and enjoy the parade of fuzzy love balls. There's nothing lonely about independence.

✔ *Share your insecurities.* It might be about work or your body, but share them with people you care about or even in a raw blog or online post. Watch how your honesty encourages others to open up.

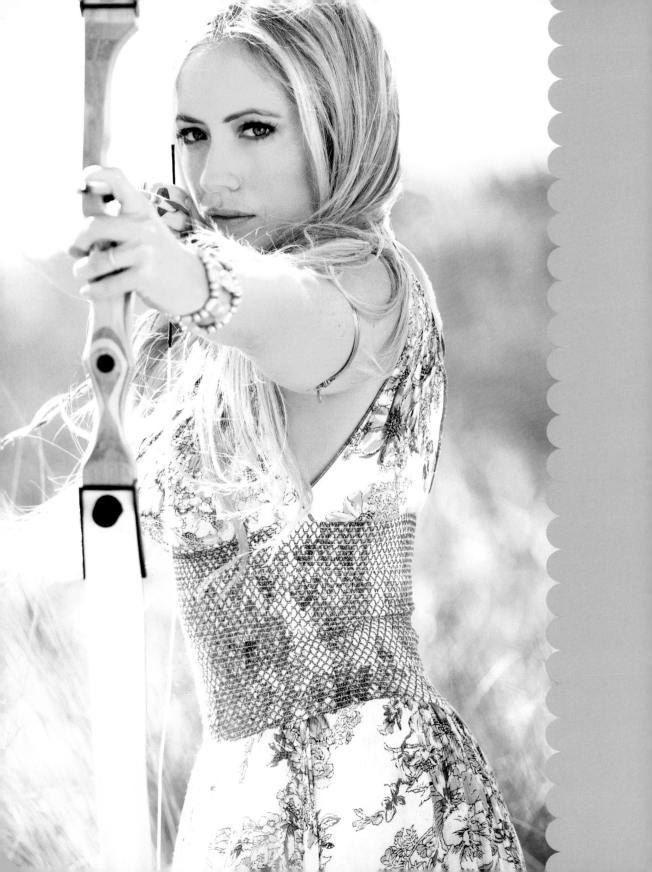

Thirteen

ALWAYS HIT *Your* MARK

It's time to challenge yourself and get way outside your comfort zone. I don't mean it's time to jump out of a plane (although I do highly recommend that, as noted in chapter 1) or take on extreme sports. I mean it's time to view failure as a part of success—they go hand in hand. They both shape and strengthen us and turn us into experienced, intelligent individuals.

Open up to all possibility and trust that the unknown is a vast place of endless potential. You don't need to know the outcome or be guaranteed success—aim true, stay true, and make your desires a reality.

One of my talents is an ability to take challenging yoga poses and make them accessible to everyone. The reason that I have the ability is because I truly wasn't very good at them in the beginning. I struggled, and because of that struggle (and constant determination to challenge myself), I became a better teacher; I can empathize with my students.

If you look at a challenging situation or person as an obstacle you couldn't possibly conquer, guess what? You're right. "No" is the most definitive sentence you can utter. The negative energy associated with disbelief is like strapping on your favorite pair of lead boots. Game over. You're going to sink all the way to the bottom and stay there.

Flip the coin and look at a challenging situation or person as what they are—indeed challenging, but certainly not impossible. You have to reach a place where you become a "yes" person—willing to tackle the unknown with a positive attitude and acceptance of success or defeat.

When you strip yourself of limiting beliefs, you give yourself the lightness to fly. No one can make things happen for you or take away the fear. You have to do that for yourself.

Pose a Challenge

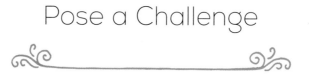

I have memories as a fledgling yogi watching third-series Ashtanga practitioners (aka very advanced) float in and out of challenging inverted and twisted postures as if they were as simple as sipping a cup of tea. These students would execute Cirque du Soleil feats as if they had the weight of a feather. I knew I wanted to experience that mobility and defiance of gravity someday, but how on earth was I going to get my lower body over my upper?

In the beginning, it wasn't pretty. I resembled a ton of bricks more than I did a floating feather. I was one of only two students in my teacher training group who couldn't kick up to handstand at the wall. I found this pose to be incredibly challenging, yet I was being stared down by a roomful of inverted eyeballs as if I were an alien. It was mortifying. Everyone kicked up, and I was flailing. My teacher sauntered over effortlessly and slid between me and the wall, using the least amount of energy to pull me up into the pose. I exhaled a sigh of gratitude and came out of the handstand flushed from more than just the pose. He smiled knowingly at me and said, "You are physically more than capable of doing this pose. It's simply when your mind is ready for it."

It struck me like a ton of yoga blocks. I still think of his words today and echo them often with my students. All poses, regardless of the challenge, are accessible to us. We simply do the work, show up with an open mind free of expectation, and do our practice. The physical body continues to grow, and as the mind frees itself, the pose arrives.

A few months later, you couldn't have peeled me out of a handstand (at the wall) if you tried. I was infused with confidence and the closest feeling to real magic.

This is why I want you to step outside of your comfort zone—to ultimately experience a delicious dose of confidence and a shot of magic into your veins. The poses that follow are difficult, no doubt, but they are all within reach. Beyond the hard work, all it takes is a willingness to be patient, open to screwing up (multiple times), and committed to enjoying the process. They are some of my favorite challenge poses— and they are just that, challenges—chosen specifically to get you going. I do recommend that you tackle them with an experienced teacher if you have the opportunity.

Choose one that intrigues you, that is outside your comfort zone, and try it. Remember to be open to all possibility, which includes struggling! Continue at it with full dedication. When your mind and physical body catch up to each other, the pose will happen—sooner or later.

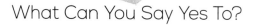

What Can You Say Yes To?

Take note of how often you say no throughout the day. Are you quick to shut down new ideas or concepts that are foreign to you? Do you find yourself saying you can't simply because you've never tried? Replace all those moments with yes. Start before you are ready, because in our minds, we never are. The time is now—embrace it with the biggest bear hug you can muster. Continue to find these examples in your life. Play the yes game and see what doors open up for you!

Will you try this new yoga pose that may mean you fall down and embarrass yourself?

You'll never grow if you never try.

Yes!

Will you come out with us tonight?

It's an opportunity to meet new tribe members, make connections—oh, and have fun.

Will you achieve that goal that you've been dreaming of for years?

This is a prime example of the power of manifestation.

Solo Challenge Poses

ADHO MUKHA VRKSASANA
(HANDSTAND)

Come into Downward-Facing Dog (page 53) with your hands shoulder width apart about 8 inches from the wall. Place the palms flat and stack the shoulders over the wrists. Rotate the triceps in and broaden the upper back. Place the shoulders in their sockets as to not tighten the base of the neck. Keep the gaze slightly forward and walk the feet in a few steps.

Lift your dominant leg, keeping the hips as square as possible. Bend the bottom knee and practice small hops, working on getting the hips over the shoulders and toward the wall. Don't worry if the legs don't go all the way up. Keep working the lift of the hips and I promise—the liftoff will come!

Once the hips get all the way over the shoulders and both feet get to the wall, let the heels rest there and flex the feet. Drive the heels up the wall to help lengthen the tailbone. Draw the frontal ribs in as you continue to hug the triceps. Firm the forearms in and keep the gaze slightly forward. Take a good 8 breaths and then take one leg away from the wall to come back into standing forward fold. Dangle and find your breath.

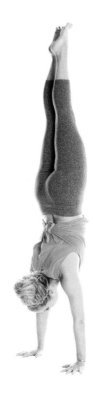

 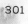

⁕ Try a Half Handstand. Come into Downward-Facing Dog with the heels pressing into where the floor and wall meet. You'll be tempted to walk your hands into a smaller Dog–don't. Keep the full stance. Work the same rotation in your arms that you created in the original instruction. Lift the right foot off the ground and take the sole of the foot a solid several feet up the wall, so it lines up with the hips. Push the sole firmly into the wall to aid the second foot in following suit. Keep the feet hip width apart and push the feet into the wall until the legs become straight. Hips will shift over the shoulders, legs are now parallel with the ground. Keep firming your arms straight, externally rotate your arms, and keep the gaze slightly past the fingertips. Hold here or practice taking one leg up at a time to get that much closer to handstand.

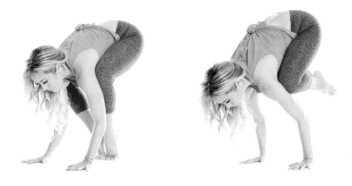

BAKASANA (CROW POSE)

Begin in a squat on the balls of your feet with your feet touching and your knees wide. Walk your hands forward, bowing your chest down so you can hug your knees with the upper outer edges of your arms. Keep squeezing your legs as you bring your hands closer to your feet and shoulder width apart. Lift your hips slightly and lean forward until you can stack your elbows over your wrists. Gaze forward and lift one foot up. Gently lean forward to pull the second foot up. Round your upper back as you press into the ground. Keep your feet tight to your hips. Hold for 5 breaths. Channel your playfulness to replace any fear or doubt. Treat this pose as a five-year-old would—as a fantastic challenge where bruises are rewarded!

VARIATION

* If face planting is a major fear, grab a pillow and place it in front of you like a crash pad. Trust me, the fall isn't that bad.
* Build a birdie perch! Place a yoga block on the lowest setting and follow the directions above from there. Practice lifting one foot at a time until you can hover your feet just above the block's surface. This additional height will give you less distance to travel and get your knees higher if your hip flexors are tight.

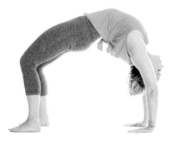

URDHVA DHANURASANA (UPWARD BOW)

Lie on your back with both knees bent and the soles of your feet on the ground hip width apart. Place your palms on the ground shoulder width apart on either side of your head. Lift your hips, press into your palms, and come up onto the crown of your head. Hug your elbows in, keep the shoulders in their sockets, and press into your hands to work your arms toward straight as you lift your body. Relax your head completely. Root into your heels to press your shinbones back (this will lift your hips) and focus on keeping your thighs and feet hip width apart. Take 8 breaths, then tuck your chin, bend your elbows, keeping them shoulder width apart, and lie down.

VARIATION

    ❊   Upward Bow is a big backbend. If you struggle with straightening your arms, just lift to the crown of your head and work on hugging your elbows in and lifting the shoulders away from the ground. Keep this up, and you'll build the strength to press up into the full pose in due time!

    ❊   For additional support, use a yoga strap. Make a lasso that measures shoulder head to shoulder head (where the bone goes into the socket). Slip this above your elbows to give you more shoulder support and prevent your arms from buckling/collapsing.

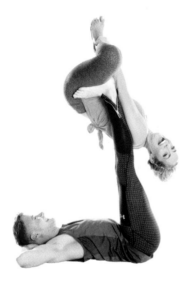

Partner and Tribe Challenge Poses

Tired of tackling fear poses as a lone wolf? Call on your pack to try a new pose together. Enjoy the support and laughter of a friend as you work toward surpassing physical or mental blocks. For each pose, designate one person as "base" and one as "flyer."

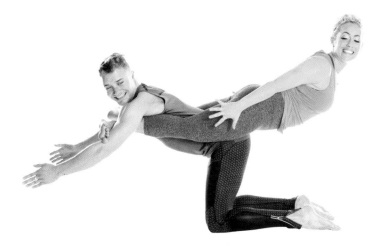

BASE: Come onto your hands and knees with your feet and knees hip width apart, as well as your hands shoulder width apart.

FLYER: Straddle your partner's hips, facing the opposite direction. Place your hands onto the ground near their feet. Hook your feet under your partner's armpits so that your toes are holding their inner arms like fingers.

BASE: Extend your arms and chest forward. Engage your core by drawing up through your lower belly.

FLYER: Extend your chest and gaze powerfully to lift your arms. Backbend your chest by drawing your shoulders back, hug your thighs powerfully around your partner's torso, and smile! You're flying!

TO EXIT: Flyer, place your hands down first, followed by Base. Flyer, unhook your feet.

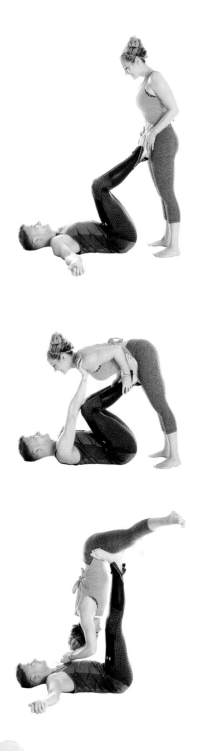

BASE: Lie on your back with your legs straight up and slightly bent.

FLYER: Stand facing your partner so that their feet can rest on your hip flexors.

BASE: With your feet hip width apart, resting on the hip flexors of your partner, your feet will naturally turn out with the shape of their pelvis. Bend your knees deeper into your chest, allowing your partner to lean toward you. Extend your arms straight, laying your hands on your partner's shoulders. As the flyer leans into your hands, extend your legs straight so they stack above your hips.

FLYER: Facing the Base, hold on to your partner's shins and lean your weight forward into their hands. Maintain eye contact as they lift you up. Let your legs straddle wide as your partner lifts you up. Spread your toes and keep the legs active. Take a moment and then let go of your partner's shins as you dangle your torso over their legs. Let your arms go limp over their chest.

BASE: Let go of your partner's shoulders once they are ready and let the flyer drape over your legs.

VARIATION:
LEAF CHEST OPENER AND TWIST

FLYER: Interlace your fingers behind your head.

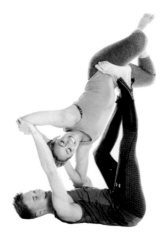

BASE: Place your hands on your partner's forearms directly below the elbows and press your arms straight to open the flyer's chest. Take a solid 5 to 8 breaths here. To twist, bend your left elbow and knee slightly as you continue to press up through your right arm and leg. Take a few breaths and switch sides.

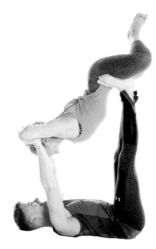

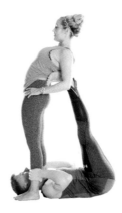

BASE: Start on your back with your legs straight up in the air.

FLYER: Straddle your feet around your partner's head facing away from them.

BASE: Grab the flyer's ankles and bring your feet to their shoulder blades.

FLYER: Melt your entire back onto your partner's feet and let your head fall back. Total surrender.

BASE: Press your feet into your partner's back until your feet stack above your hips. Simultaneously straighten your arms so they extend back at a 45-degree angle.

FLYER: Melt! You can extend your arms next to your sides, or reach them overhead and interlace all of the fingers except the index.

TO EXIT: Base, bend your elbows and knees to bring your partner's feet back to the ground where they started. Press your feet into their back to help them curl up to stand.

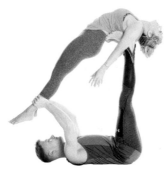

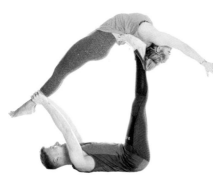

ACKNOWLEDGMENTS

I must start with a massive thank-you to the women who made this book happen—my stellar book agent, Coleen O'Shea, and my editor, Cara Bedick. You are my dream team. Thank you for believing in and understanding my vision. You are forever part of my tribe.

Deep thanks to the entire team at William Morrow/HarperCollins, especially Sharyn Rosenblum, Emily Homonoff, Molly Waxman, and Leah Carlson-Stanisic. You are a joy to work with.

Constant love for my agent and dear friend Amy Stanton, my manager Denege Prudhomme, and to the entire team at Stanton & Co., who rock my world.

I would be lost without my personal assistant, Isabel, best friend, Caroline, and the entire Shea clan. You are part of my family.

I bow down to my artistic team, who made *aim true* come to life: Cheyenne Ellis—you are a badass, a dream woman and inspiration. Lesley Unruh—you are genius and gave my recipes the sassy personalities they deserve. Cynthia Groseclose—my partner in crime, teacher, and constant source of inspiration and knowledge. Justin Schram, Kenneth Hyatt, and Nicolette Owen—your killer taste is impeccable! Elissa Genello—you just get me. We have so much beauty yet to put into the world. Sabra Mizzell—my beauty magician! Thank you for making me glow. Casey Van Zandt—you are THE stage mom extraordinaire. More thanks: Charles James, Tiffany Maloney, and Taylor Harkness.

To everyone not named who worked on set with us—thank you for the laughs and hard work.

Debbie Kim—may this be the first of many collaborations together. I have immense respect for you and your work. You are a true healer.

To my first mentor, Marty Semmelhack, who taught me the fine arts of making rice and meat sauce. To Giada De Laurentiis, for endless hours of yoga and food gab, and setting the example of what it is to be a powerful woman.

To the amazing companies who generously supported my book: Under Armour, Free People, Sage + Stone LA, Asha Patel Designs, Ox Bow Designs.

Finally, to my tribe: my friends for cheering me on; my family for always encouraging me to reach higher; my sister, Mary Frances, for being a warrior; to Bob and my four dogs, Griff, Keonah, Luna, and Ashi—I love you all to the moon and back.

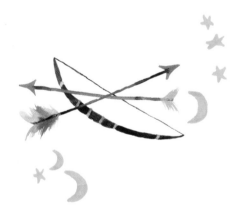

A FEW OF MY FAVORITE THINGS

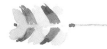

Yoga

Clothing from Under Armour Women:
www.underarmour.com

Mats from Liforme: www.liforme.com

Props from Manduka:
www.manduka.com

Websites + Apps + DVDs:

www.yogaglo.com

www.yogajournal.com

www.insighttimer.com

Aim True DVD (sold on Amazon)

Food

**Lucini Italia olive oils and San Marzano
tomatoes:** www.lucini.com

**Sun Warrior Protein Powders (the
chocolate and vanilla flavors are divine):**
www.sunwarrior.com

**Garden of Life Perfect Food Green Super
Food (the chocolate is tasty):**
www.gardenoflife.com

**Uber Greens (great with the Great Green
Monster Smoothie, page 147):**
www.pureformulas.com

**Vegenaise (my favorite vegan mayo
choice):** www.followyourheart.com

**Maldon Sea Salt Flakes (this is my sea salt
of choice):** www.maldonsalt.co.uk

**TeaPigs (liquorice and mint is my nightly
ritual):** www.teapigs.com

Kitchen

Vitamix blender: www.vitamix.com

Le Creuset cookware: www.lecreuset.com

Body

Doterra Essential Oils: www.doterra.com

Young Living Essential Oils:
www.youngliving.com

RMS Beauty: www.rmsbeauty.com

Vapour Beauty: www.vapourbeauty.com

Dr. Alkaitis: www.alkaitis.com

Éminence Organics:
www.eminenceorganics.com

Tarte Cosmetics:
www.tartecosmetics.com

Ilia Beauty: www.iliabeauty.com

UNIVERSAL CONVERSION CHART

Oven temperature equivalents

250°F = 120°C
275°F = 135°C
300°F = 150°C
325°F = 160°C
350°F = 180°C
375°F = 190°C
400°F = 200°C
425°F = 220°C
450°F = 230°C
475°F = 240°C
500°F = 260°C

Measurement equivalents

Measurements should always be level unless directed otherwise.

⅛ teaspoon = 0.5 mL
¼ teaspoon = 1 mL
½ teaspoon = 2 mL
1 teaspoon = 5 mL
1 tablespoon = 3 teaspoons = ½ fluid ounce = 15 mL
2 tablespoons = ⅛ cup = 1 fluid ounce = 30 mL
4 tablespoons = ¼ cup = 2 fluid ounces = 60 mL
5⅓ tablespoons = ⅓ cup = 3 fluid ounces = 80 mL
8 tablespoons = ½ cup = 4 fluid ounces = 120 mL
10 tablespoons = ⅔ cup = 5 fluid ounces = 160 mL
12 tablespoons = ¾ cup = 6 fluid ounces = 180 mL
16 tablespoons = 1 cup = 8 fluid ounces = 240 mL

INDEX

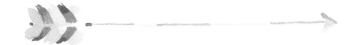

Note: Page references in *italics* indicate photographs.

ABOUT *the* AUTHOR

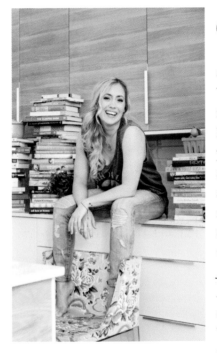

Kathryn Budig is an internationally renowned yoga teacher, author, and speaker. She was trained at Yogaworks Santa Monica by the founders, Chuck Miller and Maty Ezraty. She taught there for eight years and continues to teach and speak at conferences and workshops around the world, as well as regularly online for Yogaglo.com. She is a regular yoga and food contributor to *Women's Health, Yoga Journal, Yahoo Health,* and *Mind-BodyGreen.* She is a sponsored athlete for Under Armour's I Will What I Want campaign. Her passion for animals led her to create her nonprofit project, Poses for Paws. She resides in Charleston, South Carolina, with her husband and four dogs, Griff, Keonah, Luna, and Ashi.